BUILDING AND STRENGTHENING MUSCLES

IMPROVING HEALTH LONGEVITY AND STAYING FIT

R. F. SARMIENTO

The information herein is offered for informational purposes solely, and is universal as so. The presentation of the information is without contract or any type of guarantee assurance.

The trademarks that are used are without any consent, and the publication of the trademark is without permission or backing by the trademark owner. All trademarks and brands within this book are for clarifying purposes only and are owned by the owners themselves, not affiliated with this document.

Table Of Contents

Table Of Contents iii

INTRODUCTION 1

CHAPTER 1 WORKOUT FOR HEALTH AND FITNESS 4

ROUTINE FOR A COMPLETE BODY WORKOUT: PUSH, PULL, HINGE, SQUAT, AND CARRY 5

Routine for a Complete Body Workout 6

CHAPTER2 WORKOUT FOR HEALTH AND FITNESS 8

THE LINK BETWEEN BODYBUILDING AND FITNESS 9

MUSCLE BUILDING - REASONS WHY YOU SHOULD 11

EXERCISE AND AGEING 14

PERSONAL TRAINING - IMPROVING YOUR FITNESS INTERNALLY AND EXTERNALLY 17

THE LINK BETWEEN MUSCLE DEVELOPMENT AND NUTRITION 20

A SUITABLE BODYBUILDING DIET - REDUCE BODY FAT AND INCREASE MUSCLE 21

EXERCISES FOR BODY-BUILDING THAT WORK...... 23

CHAPTER 3 PERFECT WORKOUT AND DIET PLAN 26

HOW STRENGTHENING MUSCLE AND REDUCING FAT CAN IMPROVE YOUR HEALTH 28

The cycle of Destruction / Construction 28

MYTHS ABOUT MUSCLE BUILDING, FITNESS, AND DIET 30

THE DISTINCTION BETWEEN COMPOUND AND ISOLATION ACTIVITIES IN BODY-BUILDING EXERCISES 37

MEALS TO EAT BEFORE AND AFTER YOUR WORKOUT 38

HOW TO STRENGTHEN MUSCLE - YOUR COMPLETE, NONSENSE GUIDE 40

How to build muscle - ten quick tips! 41

CHAPTER 4 STRENGTHENING OF THE MUSCLE 48

THE BASICS OF STRENGTH TRAINING - STRENGTH TRAINING WORKOUTS AND BENEFITS 49

EXERCISES THAT STRENGTHEN THE MUSCLES 51

CAN YOU STRENGTHEN AND TONE WITHOUT A GYM? 53

Several Popular Health/Fitness Myths 57

CHAPTER 5 LEAN AND FIT PILATES 59

PILATES' SIX PRINCIPLES 60

PILATES CIRCLE - FOR STRENGTH AND FLEXIBILITY 62

STRENGTHENING OF THE CENTRAL MUSCLE 64

EXERCISES FOR CORE STRENGTHENING - THE BENEFITS 65

CORE TRAINING - SELECTING EXERCISES BASED ON STABILITY 67

TRAINING THE CORE FOR IMPROVED BODY FUNCTIONS 69

THE MOST EFFECTIVE CORE EXERCISES FOR STRENGTH AND STABILITY 70

TIPS FOR STRENGTHENING YOUR CORE MUSCLES 73

CHAPTER 6 ANTI-AGING AND VIBRATIONAL FITNESS 76

HOW DO VIBRATION PLATFORMS IMPROVE MUSCLE AND BONE STRENGTH? 78

Strength Training Benefits 80

Circulatory System Effects 82

FOR OLDER ADULTS, WHOLE-BODY VIBRATION EXERCISE AND VIBRATION TRAINING PREVENT FALLS 84

A Better Way - Drug-Free Treatment 85

The Mechanisms of Whole-Body Vibration Training and Vibration Exercise 86

A Synopsis of the Research on Vibration Exercise Machines 88

THE BIGGEST WORKOUT "MISTAKES" AND HOW TO CORRECT THEM 89

OVER- AND UNDER-TRAINING 96

CONCLUSION 99

INTRODUCTION

People frequently look at bodybuilding and say, "There is no way I could ever accomplish that." This is most likely because most of the publicity is wasted on competitors who can lift hundreds of pounds and have enormous, gigantic muscles that seem way too frightening and are the polar opposite of the muscles you want to have.

The truth is that when done correctly, bodybuilding is an excellent way to improve your health, stamina, and energy. It engages all of your muscles and helps you maintain your fitness level. When you combine bodybuilding with proper nutrition and lifestyle choices, you will have an incredible experience. Continue reading to discover some tips and strategies for mastering the art of bodybuilding.

A healthy and balanced diet should complement all bodybuilding workouts. This reduces bodybuilding to the level of any other workout. Balanced and nutritious meals are critical components of good health. This means that you should replace junk food snacks with complete grains, vegetables, and fruits.

Your adversaries are chemical additives and high fructose corn syrup. These will do nothing to improve your muscles. When you consume a natural and balanced diet, you provide your muscles with the minerals and vitamins they require to be healthy during tearing them down and rebuilding them.

Be prepared for days when your body performs less well than it normally does. Prepare to take this type of situation with stride. You should diversify your workouts and include some days of simple training to allow your muscles to recover and recuperate from the more strenuous routines you may perform.

Do not panic if your body occasionally does not perform as well as you want. Allow a day or two for rest and healing before attempting again. If you become overly stressed, you risk harm or worsening your situation.

Maintain regular contact with your physician. Your doctor can assist you in ensuring that you are getting the exercise you require while still maintaining control of your muscles. Your physician will ensure that you are not overexerting yourself, but he will also assist you in staying on track. Your doctor will assist you in identifying potential problems when they arise and ensure that they are addressed promptly before they worsen. At the absolute least, you should consult a physician before beginning the activity to ensure that your approach to bodybuilding is sound.

Bodybuilding is an excellent way to develop your strength, strengthen your muscles, and improve your general health. Many people mistakenly believe that bodybuilding is merely a recreational activity. It is an excellent way to grow, tone, and strengthen your muscles while boosting your overall health.

Maintain an optimistic attitude. The Little Engine That Could is much more than a fable for small children. This is a genuine pattern of thought. It could be the difference between your bodybuilding success and failure.

You must believe in yourself. You must maintain a good attitude, or you may become discouraged. Most significantly, if you have a happy attitude, you will achieve better bodybuilding outcomes. It's much easier to grow muscle when you're content with your actions. If you despise what you are doing, it will be more difficult for you to continue.

Bodybuilding is an entirely acceptable exercise method, increasing your strength, and improving health. Bodybuilding is frequently referred to as a "hobby" by those who do not understand it. It's an excellent approach to develop and tone your muscles while also working to improve the healthiness of your lifestyle. Body-building, when done correctly, can be an enormously satisfying technique to strengthen your entire body.

CHAPTER 1
WORKOUT FOR HEALTH AND FITNESS

The world is densely populated. Who has never known what it takes to lose weight effectively? According to them, there is only one solution: following a specific sort of diet suggested by a doctor or health specialist. They are not incorrect; they do not realize that this is only the first stage. There is a health and fitness workout if you want to achieve more lasting and rapid effects. Anyone seeking to lose weight should be prepared to participate in health and fitness activities.

Once you've created your health and fitness training routine, you must adhere to it religiously to guarantee that you maximize dieting results while also sustaining your success. If you do not plan well, the health and fitness workouts process can be difficult and ultimately fail.

You are expected to begin with what is referred to as baby steps. These are the fundamentals, and while they may appear straightforward, you must be realistic and prudent. If you visit a health and fitness professional or specialist, you will be informed that everybody's activity begins gradually and progresses over time.

Plan your health and fitness workout routine to begin with fifteen minutes of exercise and may easily repeat this practice after several days. Most individuals get it completely wrong and leave immaturely simply because they want to see results immediately. Exercise for health and fitness is a gradual procedure that should be implemented in stages.

If you believe that exercise is beneficial and body workouts are difficult and boring, crunches, push-ups, or sit-ups, you are wrong this time. You always have the option of which form of workout to participate in. Second, you can increase the enjoyment of your health and fitness workouts by exercising your favorite music. While this may appear to be a sarcastic remark, you'll notice that it produces much larger outcomes.

If you are a friendly individual at ease exercising in public, you can enroll in an aerobics class or, better yet, sessions at your local gym. While you may part with a few cents, you will benefit from working with a trained tutor. Second, you are guaranteed to make new acquaintances, because working in any group is believed to be more interesting than working alone.

A health and fitness workout does not have to take place indoors. You can also walk outside and begin jogging. If you have a track, you can always wake up and run a few kilometers in the morning. At the conclusion of the process, you will find it quite enjoyable, and even better, you will have become accustomed to it.

ROUTINE FOR A COMPLETE BODY WORKOUT: PUSH, PULL, HINGE, SQUAT, AND CARRY

Whether you're a gym rat or prefer to exercise at home, this full-body workout program has something for everyone.

It's excellent in the morning before breakfast or after work to alleviate the jitters associated with a hectic day.

In either case, sweating it out, loosening up, and incorporating every major muscle group is a straightforward weekly win.

How to Begin

Warm-up before lifting your first piece of equipment.

3 minutes jump rope (or jumping jacks)

1-minute air squat (butt to heels)

Swings of the legs: 30 seconds on each leg

Circulation of the arms: 30 seconds for each arm

Routine for a Complete Body Workout

The exercise is straightforward. Pushing, pulling, hinging, crouching, and carrying are all covered. The objective here is to make full use of your physique. This workout simulates the real world in a safe environment. Concentrate on form and repetition count.

If you cannot finish the reps with proper technique, reduce the weight. Increase your weight if you can complete the reps with enough of "gas in the tank."

The objective here is to maximize results by using your intellect and listening to your body.

That's enough jibberish... forward!

The full-body training plan consists of the following:

× 4 supersets and repetitions

Push-ups with a weighted bar - 20 reps, note: I used a 25lb plate on my back DB 12 reps bench row

12 reps deadlift

Squat with a goblet - 12 reps

Walk 30 seconds while holding a DB in one hand

60 seconds shadowbox or jump rope

30 seconds of rest

Tools

This workout will almost probably require workout equipment. Above all, you'll require a nice set of dumbbells. I prefer to perform deadlifts with a barbell, but if you do not lift high weights, the Bowflex 1090 dumbbell set is ideal.

I'm going to use the following tools for this workout:

Dumbbells

Plates for Barbell Workout

Rope jump

It would be absurd to perform this full-body workout daily. Rest is critical to exercise. If you wish to exercise the next day, take a long walk or play with your children or dogs in the yard.

And, as always, if you're unable to exercise, you can always work out in the office.

Whether or not you use these tools, make no excuses for not fitting in a quick office workout during the day.

People may laugh at you, but when you're feeling good, looking nice in the mirror, and relaxing at home, you'll be the last one to laugh!

CHAPTER2
WORKOUT FOR HEALTH AND FITNESS

The world is teeming with humanity. Who has never known what it takes to lose weight effectively? According to them, there is only one solution: following a specific sort of diet suggested by a doctor or health specialist. They are not incorrect; they do not realize that this is only the first stage. If you want to achieve more lasting and rapid effects, there is a health and fitness workout. Anyone seeking to lose weight should be prepared to participate in health and fitness activities.

Once you've created your health and fitness training routine, you must adhere to it religiously to guarantee that you maximize dieting results while also sustaining your success. If you do not plan well, the health and fitness workouts process can be difficult and ultimately fail.

You are expected to begin with what is referred to as baby steps. These are the fundamentals, and while they may appear straightforward, you must be realistic and prudent. If you visit a health and fitness professional or specialist, you will be informed that everybody's activity begins gradually and progresses over time.

Plan your health and fitness workout routine so that you begin with fifteen minutes of exercise and may easily repeat this practice after several days. Most individuals get it completely wrong and leave immaturely simply because they want to see results immediately. Exercise for health and fitness is a gradual procedure that should be implemented in stages.

If you believe that exercise and body workouts are difficult and boring crunches, push-ups, or sit-ups, you are wrong this time. You always have the option of which form of workout to participate in. Second, you can increase the enjoyment of your health and fitness workouts by exercising your favorite music. While this may appear to be a sarcastic remark, you'll notice that it produces much larger outcomes.

If you are a friendly individual at ease exercising in public, you can enroll in an aerobics class or, better yet, sessions at your local gym. While you may part with a few cents, you will benefit from working with a trained tutor. Second, you are guaranteed to make new acquaintances, because working in any group is believed to be more interesting than working alone.

A health and fitness workout does not have to take place indoors. You can also walk outside and begin jogging. If you have a track, you can always wake up and run a few kilometers in the morning. At the conclusion of the process, you will find it quite enjoyable, and even better, you will have become accustomed to it.

THE LINK BETWEEN BODYBUILDING AND FITNESS

Bodybuilding enthusiasts are well aware of the effort required to develop and maintain the sculpted bodies they aspire to. A structured diet is undoubtedly a significant component of bodybuilding - reducing fat and increasing lean protein to fuel the body's muscles and maximize nutrition. However, the link between bodybuilding and fitness is apparent when it comes to acquiring the ideal physique desired by most bodybuilders.

Bodybuilding and fitness are inextricably linked because intense and consistent workouts mostly determine muscular mass. Bodybuilders will tell you how many hours they spend in the gym performing cardiovascular exercises, stretching, and significant weight training. This training is critical for those competing. Any competitor will tell you that bodybuilding and fitness are inextricably linked; one cannot exist without the other.

Little steps must be taken to build up a comprehensive training regimen for many new people in bodybuilding and fitness. It is critical to balance cardio with core and weight training to reach peak fitness. Cardiovascular exercise can take the form of running, walking, dancing, and kickboxing. Following, intensive core training such as Pilates or yoga will strengthen abdominal muscles, improve flexibility, and keep muscles limber.

But when it comes to bodybuilding and fitness, nothing works more to grow and retain muscle mass than weight training. Whether using weight training machines or free weights, lifting weights - when done correctly - will augment and shape muscular mass throughout the body. Bodybuilders rely on weight training to reach their fitness goals.

However, it is extremely crucial that if you don't have expertise with weight training, you get professional coaching to master the appropriate techniques. Weights, when lifted wrongly, will only serve to harm rather than develop muscles.

People wishing to develop their bodies and perhaps compete in bodybuilding competitions need to adopt a constant nutrition and exercise schedule in their lives. For this reason, bodybuilding and fitness will continue to be an inseparable and permanent combo.

MUSCLE BUILDING - REASONS WHY YOU SHOULD

Have you ever met a bodybuilder? and thought to yourself, "Why did he bother to build all those muscles?" For the bodybuilder, the answer may have to do with overcoming adversity or experiencing the rush of competition. However, there are numerous reasons why everyone should want to increase their muscular mass through strength exercise. This essay will discuss seven of the most compelling reasons to grow muscle.

1. Improve Your Mood

If you've been feeling sad recently, an exercise incorporating strength training can help you feel better.

Have you ever pondered why fitness instructors often appear to be a little too optimistic? This is because physical activity makes people happy. Exercise has been demonstrated to boost one's mood. Indeed, many physicians who treat people suffering from depression advocate exercise as a component of treatment.

Therefore, begin a strength training plan and you should begin to feel better shortly.

2. Enhance Your Appearance

You will feel better after beginning a strength training program, but you will also notice an improvement in your appearance. Regardless of whether you're a man or a woman, your physical attractiveness will improve as you grow muscle.

Let's be honest; muscle is more appealing than fat. When you visit the beach or a swimming pool, you will appear better in your swimwear. Your clothes will fit you better.

And don't forget about the effect on the opposite sex. If you're single and having difficulty finding dates, increasing your lean muscle mass will also help you enhance your dating prospects.

3. Increased Strength

While it may seem self-evident that growing muscle will make you stronger, many people underestimate the value of improved strength.

If you've ever had difficulty opening a jar of pickles or need assistance moving a box of books, you realize the constraints that diminished strength may have on your life.

A strength training plan can considerably increase your strength and enable you to perform various tasks requiring assistance.

4. Boosted Metabolism

Your body's muscle cells consume energy, whereas fat cells store it. Thus, increasing muscle mass through strength training increases your body's energy requirements. This speeds up your metabolism, causing your body to burn more fat.

Therefore, if you've been battling to shed excess body fat over the years, begin a new strength training regimen. The additional lean muscle mass you get will make it much easier to reduce excess fat.

5. Increased Self-Belief

Individuals who exercise regularly have a greater sense of self-confidence than those who do not. If you struggle with self-confidence, strength training can assist.

Muscle development can boost your confidence in a variety of ways. To begin, a more positive self-image. As you begin to replace body fat with lean muscle, you will notice an improvement in your appearance in the mirror. This will significantly improve your self-esteem and provide you with the confidence you require in other areas of your life.

Second, as you begin to transform your body, you will attract the attention of others. They will begin to show you greater respect. This will become apparent to you, consciously or subconsciously, and profoundly affect your self-confidence.

Third, simply setting and attaining goals can boost your confidence. Therefore, set a goal to begin strength training today, and you will quickly see an increase in your self-confidence.

6. Avoid Injuries

Strength training can aid in the prevention of a variety of injuries.

By strengthening your core, you can enhance your balance and coordination and decrease your risk of being injured in an accident.

Muscle development also strengthens and grows your bones and tendons, which can help avoid fractured bones and tendon strains and tears. Modern athletes in various sports use muscle training to assist them in improving athletically and reducing the occurrence of injuries.

It is critical to maintaining our muscular training routines as we age to avoid the injuries that senior people are prone to.

7. Enhancement of overall health and fitness

Strength training improves your fitness and conditioning levels, which greatly affects your overall health.

Individuals who regularly engage in moderate physical activity have a reduced disease risk. Then those who are sedentary. Weight training has been found to lessen the risk of heart disease by increasing cardiovascular function and blood chemistry.

After reading these seven reasons to begin muscle building, you're probably ready to shut off your computer and head to the gym. Remember to begin slowly and consult your physician before beginning any new workout program.

EXERCISE AND AGEING

You do not have to disintegrate as you age - it is possible to halt or reverse the aging process. Our bodies undergo morphological and physiological changes when we approach 50. Through regular physical activity, we can halt or reverse these effects.

The Thoughts and Exercises of Joseph Pilates

According to Joseph Pilates, "The spine was critical to physical and mental health. The importance of neutral spine alignment cannot be overstated." He said, " "At 30, if your spine is stiff, you are ancient. If it is malleable at the age of 60, you are still young."

Pilates exercise strengthens the back and abdomen muscles that support the spine. Numerous people, including myself, can follow his exercise regimen. It offers significant health benefits as we age.

He was a man who was decades ahead of his time. On a worldwide basis, it is only in the last 25 years that we have truly embraced his ideas. His fitness regimen paves the path for elderly adults to enjoy their later years. It can increase your overall mobility dramatically—strength and posture long into your 80s and beyond.

If you watch some films of Joseph Pilates exercising in his final years on YouTube, you will be in awe of his athleticism and mobility.

Neuromuscular Alterations

Reduced testosterone production

Muscle atrophy, particularly fast-twitch muscle

With age, connective tissues become less elastic.

In our thirties, we are at our strongest and most powerful. This trend continues into our fifties.

Following this, we lose approximately 10 oz of muscle mass per year. Men and women alike who reach the age of 70. will have lost 40% of their muscle mass. Does that sound frightening?

This muscle loss is partly related to decreased testosterone production. Muscle loss also includes fast-twitch muscle fibers (muscles used for quick movement). Falling risk is associated with diminished fast-twitch muscle and total muscular loss in the elderly.

Additionally, connective tissue loses its elasticity as people age, which explains why many older adults complain of muscle stiffness.

Resistance workouts for seniors maintain or improve muscle strength, suppleness, and mass.

Composition of the Body

As we age, muscular mass decreases, and body fat increases. As previously stated, this drop in muscle mass is caused by decreased testosterone production. Due to the fact that muscle consumes more calories than fat, the combination of muscle loss and fat gain decreases your metabolic rate.

Muscle mass can be increased by aerobic and resistance training. Muscles burn fat following resistance training to rebuild and strengthen themselves. This is the area where fat is lost. By performing these workouts, you can halt the onset of fat gain.

Dietary changes can also help you maintain healthy body composition. Increased protein intake in conjunction with decreased carbohydrate intake will aid in the maintenance of muscle mass and the reduction of body fat. Unless you decrease your calorie intake as you age, you will acquire weight naturally in the form of fat.

The posture of the Body

Our bodies deteriorate as we age. Known as 'Kyphosis,' this condition causes the shoulders to curve and the head forward.

Weight-bearing exercise or resistance training helps maintain the strength of the skeletal and muscular systems, which helps keep the back in the proper position for proper body posture.

Gait

This is the term used to refer to our walking style. Speed and stride length diminishes with age. The pelvis can be shifted, and ankle movement restricted.

Core strength training strengthens the abdominal muscles, hence reversing the pelvic tilt.

Regular mobility exercises help preserve ankle mobility.

Aerobic exercise at a moderate intensity maintains a healthy stride length and frequency.

It is entirely possible to remain healthy and strong into your 80s and beyond. The most prudent method to begin a fitness program, particularly if you are new to exercise, is to talk with a certified gym instructor or personal trainer.

They will examine your present state of health and fitness before designing a program just for you. As your strength and fitness levels improve, your trainer will increase the intensity of your aerobic and resistance activities. Not to fear; your fitness teacher will oversee your training program to ensure safety and progress.

PERSONAL TRAINING - IMPROVING YOUR FITNESS INTERNALLY AND EXTERNALLY

Physical activity performed in moderation is ideal for personal training that benefits the physical and mind and heart. It is a wonderful alternative for individuals who want to look and feel their best.

Proper personal training entails a sound physical regimen and sound nutrition, adequate sleep, and an overall wholesome way of life. Swimming, walking, running, cycling, or tennis are excellent ways to spend your time. Are all cardiovascular exercises. Flexibility activities such as stretching, contracting, and other types of flexibility exercises help to strengthen muscles and joints. Lifting weights, sprinting, and other functional exercises focus on short-term muscle gain and strengthening.

Consider the benefits of personal training on the body.

For the Physical Physique

Muscles, bones, and joints make up most of the human body. Muscles give the body its form and shape. While bones are designed to support weight, joints allow the body to move. Physical activity contributes to developing and maintaining muscle strength, healthy bone density, and joint mobility. Exercise increases the body's energy level, which is required for daily physical activity such as traveling, performing home tasks, or exercising your career.

Regular physical activity aids with weight management. Excess weight is frequently related to excess fat in the body, resulting in diabetes and other chronic cardiac illnesses. Excessive body weight impairs people's ability to sleep, breathe, walk, run, and maneuver. Overweight and obese individuals frequently experience discomfort due to their appearance, decreasing their self-image and self-esteem.

Proper exercise oxygenates and nourishes the body's tissues. Healthy bodily tissues provide a robust immune system and aid in the battle against certain chronic health diseases such as diabetes, hypertension, respiratory tract infections, and some kinds of breast and colon cancer.

For the Soul

The heart gets more powerful and efficient at transporting blood to all body regions with regular physical activity. The blood arteries are strengthened, which improves circulation. Blood cholesterol levels are brought down, hence lowering the risk of stroke. Thirty minutes of moderate aerobic activity five times a week or 20 minutes of intense exercise three times a week, depending on your health status and age, is an effective program for maintaining a healthy heart.

For the Mind

The brain is composed of nerve cells known as neurons that transmit electrical signals. These impulses are in charge of instructing the body on what to perform. If you wish to make a movement with your finger, the neurons guide the impulses to the finger.

Regular physical activity contributes to the generation of neurons. Additionally, physical activity has improved memory and eases both mental and physical pain. Regular exercisers are more wise, intuitive, and joyful.

Moderation and consistency are critical components of a sustainable personal training program. Excessive exercise, like excessive eating and sleep, is hazardous to your health. Excessively rigorous activity can cause muscle damage, bone fractures, joint sprains, and overwork of the heart and brain.

A healthy level of physical activity is both enjoyable and not exhausting. You should now be prepared to walk, run, swim, or dance to look and feel beautiful on the inside and out.

THE LINK BETWEEN MUSCLE DEVELOPMENT AND NUTRITION

Whether or not you exercise, a balanced diet is critical. However, diet becomes crucial as muscle-building routines if you want to sculpt your body through exercise.

You are mistaken if you believe that nutrition is about bingeing on green vegetables. Nutrition is the consumption of a balanced diet that contains all of the nutrients necessary for Body-building, from vitamins and minerals to fats and proteins.

When training to gain muscle mass, you require at least 40 more calories per kilogram of body weight each day. These additional calories provide the energy required to complete the intense training. Additionally, this does not mean you may overindulge in junk food following your workouts!

However, you must create your food plan or ask your teacher to do so for you to get the proper nutrients. Proteins are the most critical aspect of diet, as they are the building blocks of muscles. To heal injured muscles and grow new ones, it is critical to consume somewhat more protein in your diet.

Carbohydrates and lipids in moderation are essential for exercise energy. Muscle development requires at least 50% of calories to come from carbohydrates to build glycogen, the body's primary source of energy. The healing of tissue and developing core strength and stamina requires minerals and vitamins found in fresh fruits and vegetables.

Calcium, zinc, and iron are essential for bone strength and blood formation. Having a complete food plan that takes your nutrition into account is critical for muscular growth. Additionally, you can use bio-organic supplement shakes such as Shakeology, which has over 70 essential nutrients to help you stay energized and healthy.

A SUITABLE BODYBUILDING DIET - REDUCE BODY FAT AND INCREASE MUSCLE

Diet and nutrition are critical components of a successful bodybuilding regimen and will determine your level of achievement. Without sufficient nourishment, training is like swimming upstream. All of your training will be in vain.

A decent bodybuilding diet must adhere to three rules:

1. Consume smaller portions throughout the day.
2. Each meal should contain carbohydrates, protein, and fat: 40% carbs, 40% protein, and 20% healthy fats.
3. Calorie consumption should be cycled to avoid erroneous metabolism.

It is vital to restrict certain foods and include a variety of nutrient-dense foods in your regular diet when following a muscle-building diet. If your goal is to develop into a lean muscle man or woman, you must ensure that you feed the proper type of body mass transformation. Several dietary ideas for developing a fit and excellent muscular body include the following:

Consumption of Lean Meat-Lean meats is high in protein, which the body requires to create muscle strength. Pork, beef, and goat meat are high in protein.

Even poultry feed and fish provide a plethora of nutritional benefits. They are a staple of many-body builders' diets throughout the world. However, avoid oily and fatty foods in your diet. It is preferable to roast, boil, or grill your meal rather than fry it.

Foods high in fiber-Fibers are a wonderful choice for individuals looking to lose weight. Foods high in fiber prevent the body from absorbing fat. It helps maintain a healthy body cholesterol level.

Because fiber is indigestible, it takes a long time to break down into carbohydrates. Numerous fiber-rich foods are available, including oats, wheat germ, spinach, fresh fruits, and cereals.

Supplements to supplement your bodybuilding regimen are readily available in various health stores.

Liquid Intake-Water is the most critical liquid supply for a bodybuilder, as activity depletes the body's natural fluids. Consuming plenty of water is critical for maintaining a healthy energy level and body temperature.

Soybeans—Because they are high in protein, they are low in fat. They contain no cholesterol, making them a perfect diet for fitness enthusiasts.

Soybean is claimed to increase muscle strength and help you lose weight. Soybeans are found in tofu, curds, beans, and various desserts.

Whey protein-Whey proteins are readily available at most health clinics and retail locations. It is versatile and may be paired with soups, smoothies, and cooked veggies. Additionally, it can be used as a supplement. It is gentle on the body due to its ease of digestion and is one of the highest protein-containing foods available.

Eggs-Eggs, particularly egg whites, are a good source of protein. However, it is preferable to avoid the egg yolk. In health food stores, processed egg whites are accessible.

To build lean muscle mass, you must combine an adequate calorie intake with a rigorous muscular strengthening regimen. Calories are required to fuel both workouts and tissue growth. Utilize this knowledge to assist you in developing a bodybuilding diet.

EXERCISES FOR BODY-BUILDING THAT WORK

Before beginning any muscle-building workout program, there are a few critical points to remember, most of which pertain to optimizing the benefits obtained when the activity is planned and executed properly. Unfortunately, most people who begin muscle development programs end up cheating because they do not devote sufficient time to mastering the proper exercises for a successful muscle-building regimen during the initial stages. Here is some sound advice. That can help you achieve more success in general.

Most muscle-building trainers can guide beginners and seasoned muscle builders on the right route. Because they have the expertise to assist individuals in selecting the ideal workouts for their unique goals and objectives, they can significantly increase their results.

For example, when a professional trainer assists an individual in selecting a customizable exercise plan, they typically recommend one that will prevent them from wasting unnecessary time and effort in the gym, which means they will typically recommend a program that will effectively build lean muscle mass while also increasing testosterone levels in the body. When done correctly, the individual will lose fat and enjoy a bigger amplitude of post-workout outcomes, which will enhance their muscle-building rate.

Here's a quick overview of the finest muscle-building exercises and how they influence the various body regions.

Squats - Squats are exercises that emphasize the lower body. Thus, when performed properly, they concentrate on strengthening and growing the glutes, core, quads, hamstrings, and spinal column.

Split Squats - Once an individual has mastered the proper technique for performing conventional squats, they should focus on split squats as their next exercise. These workouts are oriented for glute-building and core strengthening, as they must be completed in an off-balance position.

Deadlifts and muscle-building exercises are typically performed when individuals concentrate on developing a more defined buttock, strengthening their lower back muscles, and increasing their glute muscular strength.

Pull-Ups - When someone performs pull-ups, they should at the very least understand why they are so effective. While they are designed to stabilize the entire body, they also give an excellent exercise for the core, biceps, and lat muscles.

Push-Ups - Push-Ups is typically a challenging workout to perfect for both men and women. However, when carried out properly, individuals can attain maximum outcomes.

Additionally, because push-ups may be performed in various ways and permutations, they prevent individuals from becoming bored soon. These workouts are also beneficial for strengthening the individual's chest, biceps, and triceps.

Lunges - Lunges are also a staple of many muscle-building programs. Specifically, they may be performed with barbells and dumbells, which helps to increase their effectiveness. Lunges are often accomplished by crossing these sets (dumbells or barbells) over the back with the correct body movement.

Step-Ups - When people incorporate step-ups into their fitness routine, they frequently discover how versatile they are. Because these exercises can be regarded as a lower body workout that aids in fat loss, most women like including them in their regular routines; step-ups can be used to increase muscle and improve agility.

Shoulder Press - Another excellent technique to maintain upper body strength is to do shoulder press workouts. This exercise is beneficial because it strengthens the key shoulder joints and contributes significantly to upper body strength.

Bent-Over Rows - Bent-over rows are the ideal workout for strengthening the back muscles. For individuals unfamiliar with how these are executed, they may wish to picture shoulder blade squeezing movements.

Bench Press - The bench press is a widespread and popular exercise used to build muscle in various body areas, including the triceps, chest, shoulders, and biceps.

CHAPTER 3
PERFECT WORKOUT AND DIET PLAN

Working out or participating in inactivity has become an integral aspect of an individual's fitness and health program. It is used in conjunction with a diet food plan to help you obtain a more attractive body shape and maintain optimal health. It strengthens and improves muscular structure, burns fat, and increases strength, contributing to overall wellness and self-confidence.

Maintaining a diet compatible with your workout routine may appear to be difficult. You're unsure whether you should eat more or less? Additionally, you'll be thinking about what foods you're going to consume that won't negate or diminish the effects of your workout.

Before an hour and a half (90 minutes) and after your workout and an hour (60 minutes), it is a key time to consume foods that encourage peak productivity and performance. This is known as the four-hour window. Thus, we must consume the proper foods throughout these periods.

Plans/tricks for pre-workout diets:

During your workout, your body will eat your stored glucose or sugar and convert it to the energy (ATP) required. As a result, consumption is crucial. Carbohydrates before exercising. This will ensure that adequate and readily available nutrients are consumed to maximize training potential. Additionally, it is recommended to consume adequate fluids (about 17 oz) because your body will lose fluids through sweat during energy conversion.

A substantial lunch should be consumed three to four hours before the activity, while a light snack should be consumed an hour before. Simple carbs, such as juices and fruits, are good for providing an immediate energy supply to the body. Low-glycemic carbohydrate sources such as yogurt and skimmed milk aid in fat burning. Proteins are also important for exercise-related strength.

Plans/tricks for post-workout diets:

After your workout, you should eat as quickly as possible (about 30 minutes to an hour); it is critical to replenish what you have lost. Proteins increase endurance by forming new or repairing damaged tissues, and they can act as a source of energy if your carbohydrate and lipid stores or resources are depleted. Thus, you must consume protein following your workout.

Along with protein, you must need carbohydrates. Simple carbohydrate and protein sources are chosen over-complicated carbohydrate and protein sources because they are quickly digested and do not decrease metabolism. Additionally, it is critical to avoid fats following a workout because they impede digestion, interfering with the necessary carbohydrate and protein digestion. Finally, do not forget to hydrate yourself.

Simply take this simple step to ensure that your workout and food plans are in sync and that you achieve the greatest possible results.

HOW STRENGTHENING MUSCLE AND REDUCING FAT CAN IMPROVE YOUR HEALTH

Every person's health objective should be to gain muscle and strength. It contains many beneficial characteristics, some readily apparent and some of which are not. Your sleek, defined figure will help you fight sickness and strengthen your heart, lungs, and other essential organs. Weight training properly results in beneficial muscular increases. If you are sedentary and begin a fat loss program, your body will respond swiftly if the physical fitness routines are applied consistently.

If your job requires physical exertion, which requires frequent lifting of big objects, constant strength training will enable you to safely do your work and avoid injury. A muscular person is significantly more capable of completing a day's job with energy to spare. Let's examine how muscular development benefits your health and fitness.

The cycle of Destruction / Construction

The human body is a self-healing mechanism. It operates similarly to a city, with all of its departments responsible for the day-to-day operations of critical services. It delivers nutrients necessary for system maintenance and waste necessary for system protection. When a component fails, its engineers labor quickly to repair the damage and strengthen the afflicted area against future damage.

Thus, your body heals and strengthens whenever you subject your muscles to significant stress through intense exercise. It's as if city planners and engineers collaborate to prioritize problem areas for improvement in preparation for future failures.

Not only is the impacted area upgraded, but also the distribution system. Increased blood flow throughout the body facilitates more oxygen delivery to your muscles. As a result, they grow faster and stronger following each tough session. With each incremental session, this increased blood flow lessens your degree of weariness.

Consider the basic act of executing pull-ups. If you begin with none, you will continue to work on it until you can perform one pull-up. To accomplish this, your body must compensate for external stress and gradually grow muscles dedicated to the goal of lifting your body off the ground. This may be a little accomplishment, but shortly after your initial success, your body will have acclimated to the effort and be prepared to build up to two pull-ups.

Muscle building is a progressive process that entails destroying muscles at the cellular level and allowing the body to rebuild them. Progressive load-bearing refers to increasing the number of reps, sets, or weights in an activity to compensate for the body's ability to adapt. Gradually raising the load helps your muscles develop and protects you from harm caused by inappropriate weight use.

The remaining two jigsaw pieces are dietary support and sufficient healing. It is also critical to nourish the injured cells and allow them time to repair to become stronger and more elastic.

MYTHS ABOUT MUSCLE BUILDING, FITNESS, AND DIET

MYTH 1 >>Strength training Transforms Females Into Males.

TRUE: This fallacy is especially prevalent among women, who fear that lifting weights will bulk them out. If you compared a pound of fat and a pound of muscle side by side, you'd note that the muscle is smaller despite being the same weight.

Which debunks another myth: muscle is heavier than fat. One pound of muscle always weighs the same as 1 pound of fat.

The more muscle you have, the less space you will require.

Women are unable to bulk up by lifting high weights. Ladies' hormone profiles contain an excess of estrogen. While bigger weights help build muscle and strength, most women are not lifting anything nearly as heavy as the Incredible Hulk. Additionally, muscle is the key to a boosted metabolism, as it burns more calories than fat, even while sitting on the sofa or at your desk.

Thus, the trend for women to lift lighter weights and perform more reps than males is irresponsible. Women cannot accomplish exceptional muscle growth without the use of chemicals. Because women's testosterone levels are lower than men's, they will likely be unable to lift as much weight as men. Still, the standard three-pound lady dumbbells will not work because the resistance is insufficient to produce muscular change.

Why do women develop muscles if they are not intended to? While the notion of "manly" varies by everyone, we all have a unique body structure. Some women have more feminine features, while others have more androgynous features. Although broad hip bones and small shoulders are traditional female shapes, an athletic lady is no less feminine. Our society shapes our ideals; you choose what appeals to you.

Sporty women bulky is a greater than usual muscular mass and "extra" body fat. If you combine weight exercise with a sensible diet, you will lose far more weight than you think.

The basic line is that strength training can aid with weight loss. More quickly and keep it off. If you incorporate cardio into your workout plan, you'll preserve muscle while losing fat and prevent your metabolism from decreasing.

MYTH 2>>I am capable of resolving my issues on a case-by-case basis

TRUTII: Spot reduction is impossible unless surgery is performed. Without it, your body will take fat from various locations at varying rates based on your genetic makeup. Rather than concentrating on a single location, spend your time engaging in full-body workouts that burn calories.

This is also true for six-packs or a flat stomach.

You can perform crunches until you pass out and yet not achieve a six-pack. Save yourself the effort and potential back strain by recognizing that the best method to achieve a six-pack is improved nutritional choices and high-intensity interval training.

Every person is born with abdominal muscles. You simply need to shed fat for them to shine out.

MYTH 3>>Carbohydrates Are Your Enemy

THE TRUTH: The only way to lose the appropriate weight is to eat a balanced diet that supports your goal, train weights, and incorporate cardio. Your program should incorporate all of these components for an extended period to observe a difference.

Diet, weight training, and cardio-the fitness holy trifecta!

Carbohydrates are required for muscle growth. If you eliminate them, you will likely burn more body fat during exercising, but this will not last long. Carbohydrates provide fuel for strenuous workouts, while fats do not.

Carbohydrates, protein, and fat are the macronutrients required for a well-balanced nutritional regimen. All three of these are vital and play critical roles in the body. I will not detail this here since a comprehensive discussion of macronutrients and their functions would be lengthy. They would be addressed more correctly. In a separate post. On nutrition that I will publish later.

The simplest way to phrase this fallacy is: "How much carbs do you consume and when?" Whole grains, legumes, veggies, and minimally processed grains are all excellent sources of carbohydrates that you can regularly have.

MYTH 4>>The Only Way to Lose Weight Is to Run

TRUTH: Your fitness achievement is contingent upon your objective. If you want to run 10 miles without breaking a sweat, you must run.

If you aim to reduce fat or increase muscle, incorporating cardio and weight training into your program is the most efficient method.

Weight training is essential for maintaining our upright, aligned, and powerful posture. The ultimate goal of preventing our bodies from collapsing as we age is to raise the arches of our feet, strengthen our pelvic floor, and keep our heads from going forward.

Strengthens tendons and ligaments while also increasing bone density. While cardio is beneficial for bone density and is necessary for maintaining a healthy heart, it does not keep your body in alignment or build your major postural muscles. Maintain a healthy balance and include weight training and cardio in your routine.

MYTH No. 5>> Exercise is most beneficial in the morning.

TRUTH: Unless you are a professional athlete who trains twice or three times a day, there is no optimal time to exercise.

The optimal timing is convenient for you and fits into your schedule.

By listening to your body and determining when you perform best, you can determine whether mornings, afternoons, or nighttime workouts are, in fact, your time of power. Energy and attitude are critical components of effective training. Therefore, become familiar with your body clock and attempt to go to the gym when you are at your strongest.

MYTH NO. 6>> Without discomfort, there is no gain.

TRUTH: Results, not soreness, indicate a successful workout. The localized muscular ache that subsides after a few days shows that you worked hard. To build strength and endurance, you may need to endure a mild level of discomfort.

of discomfort; however, this is not the same as pain. "No pain, no gain" is not an effective strategy for creating a lifelong exercise regimen.

Soreness is the result of inflammation and the chemical response to it. The sole metric that must be used to gauge your success is that of your goal. Assess your workout based on what occurs during it.

MYTH NO. 7>> The most effective strategy to lose weight is dramatically reducing your calorie intake.

TRUTH: Our bodies are more intelligent than we believe. When we eat insufficiently, our bodies assume they are starving, and as a result, our metabolism slows, and fat is stored as a possible energy source.

When some people attempt diets, more than 90% of those who lose weight through dieting regain it.

Dieting for a fast fix is not the same as changing your eating habits.

Eating healthfully entails acquiring a new mindset. The genuine weight-loss formula is a lifetime of moderate activity.

MYTH 8>>If you want to lose weight, you must abstain from fat.

TRUTH: Fats must maintain normal hormone levels and utilize vitamins properly. Without it, you'll create an atmosphere detrimental to muscle growth. Additionally, fats aid with appetite regulation. A carbohydrate- and protein-only diet can make achieving any fat-loss or muscle-building objective impossible.

Healthy fats such as avocados, almonds, peanut butter, and olive oil are "clean" and can aid in weight loss. However, even a completely clean diet does not guarantee weight loss. You can be obese while eating only "clean" foods.

MYTH 9>>If You Train Hard Enough, You Can Eat Anything

TRUE: A poor diet cannot be out-trained.

You must spend more calories than your body consumes to burn fat. You cannot expect to sit around all day eating hamburgers and assume that a few workouts a week will help you lose weight. That is a ridiculous remark.

MYTH 10>> The more sweat you generate, the more fat you lose.

TRUTH: Sweating has nothing to do with intensity; it is simply your body's method of removing heat. Within your body, fat is oxidized, and it will not vaporize due to your sweat!

MYTH 11>> Fruit is a fat-free snack.

TRUTH: We consume food to obtain nutrients and energy, yet any food, regardless of its nutritional value, can cause weight gain. Fruit contains a high concentration of carbohydrates that are quickly absorbed. By providing your body with readily available carbohydrates, you effectively tell it to stop utilizing body fat for fuel.

Additionally, the fruit has a high proportion of fructose stored in the liver rather than muscles. Additionally, loading up on high-calorie fruit will fail to reach your fat-loss objective.

Compared to fruit, vegetables include more minerals, vitamins, and even anti-cancer qualities. The calorie composition of the two dietary groups differs. Vegetables are generally lower in calories than fruit.

MYTH 12>> After 40, it is impossible to grow muscle.

TRUTH: While age can cause wear and tear if you've been a competitive professional athlete since a teenager, you're still a training baby at 40. Our metabolism slows down as we age Due to decreased hormone levels and decreased physical activity. At any age, you can develop muscle. As long as you continue, your body will respond. To challenge your muscles and provide them with the necessary nutrition. Muscle growth becomes more difficult as we age.

However, as with anything, if you give it your all, you will succeed.

THE DISTINCTION BETWEEN COMPOUND AND ISOLATION ACTIVITIES IN BODY-BUILDING EXERCISES

There are numerous exercises, and each of these workouts can be performed in various ways, including with free weights, machines, gadgets, or your body weight resistance, among others. Some argue that isolation exercises should be used more than compound workouts, while others argue that the reverse is true.

Both are right to a point, and it all depends on the objective or style of training. For bodybuilding, isolation and complex exercises are the two fundamental types of exercises, and both should be performed in training to maximize overall muscle activation and growth.

The distinction is as follows:

Isolation exercises concentrate on a particular muscle and typically involve only one joint action, such as leg extensions and bicep curls.

Compound exercises involve the engagement of two or more muscles and the movement of multiple joints, such as squats, which involve the movement of your knees and hip joints, and bench presses.

What is the purpose of each?

Muscle builders utilize isolation workouts to strengthen or improve the growth of a muscle. As you continue to execute Body-building workouts consistently, you may notice that your right bicep needs some shaping to balance out its strength or size compared to your left bicep. Next, you would isolate that muscle by completing a dumbbell preacher curl for your right bicep muscle, an isolation exercise.

Compound workouts are primarily utilized to increase general strength and muscle growth from a muscle-building standpoint. A single exercise requires the utilization of multiple muscle groups to lift the weight, and the larger muscles are often the ones responsible.

Compound workouts enable you to lift significantly more weight. With the assistance of many muscles, they result in the rapid growth of overall mass. Additionally, these workouts are a natural approach for individuals to lift, push, and pull objects. Consider this: When you move a somewhat heavier box from one location to another, you rely on your leg, back, and arm muscles to complete the work.

As you can see, both compound and isolation workouts contribute to the overall effectiveness of your workout. You can increase your strength and general muscular mass by performing rigorous compound exercises and then using isolation workouts to shape muscles that were not fully utilized during your compound activities.

Incorporating both sorts of exercises into your bodybuilding workouts is the way to go, as long as the combination is appropriate for your unique demands. And when executed well, it can make a significant difference.

MEALS TO EAT BEFORE AND AFTER YOUR WORKOUT

You probably know that the most effective method for losing extra fat and increasing muscle mass is to adhere to a healthy eating and exercise regimen. However, you may not realize that your exercise efforts may be futile unless you pay close attention to your pre-and post-workout meals. Indeed, the two most vital meals of the day are consumed around an hour before and after a training session. It can mean the difference between improving your body's inherent capacity for muscle growth and squandering your gym time.

Pre-workout meals are designed to prime your body for the massive pressure and stress it will shortly face. When your body depletes its stored energy during strenuous activities, it begins converting carbs into the energy required to contract your muscles. Therefore, it is only normal for you to consume carbohydrates before a training session to ensure that Your body contains the required nutrients. To produce energy.

To enhance your body's muscle-building potential, pre-workout meals should be primarily complex carbohydrates and proteins. Ensure that your body has sufficient time to assimilate these nutrients and that they are easily available. At the same time, you exercise; it is ideal for eating at least one hour before your training session. Additionally, you can take a protein shake. Or fresh fruit juice supplemented with protein powder 15 minutes before your activity.

The most critical meals of the day are post-workout. Remember that a hard training session frequently results in micro-tears in your muscles, which your body will naturally strive to mend and strengthen in the hours following the activity. To ensure that your muscles can truly repair, you must consume the appropriate post-workout foods.

Carbohydrates are required for fuel replenishment, whereas protein is required for muscle repair and strengthening. Consume these nutrients as soon as possible so that your body can begin mending itself. Therefore, post-workout meals aim to immediately refuel your body and supply it with necessary nutrients for muscle repair and strengthening.

A sports drink is a wonderful way to kick-start your post-workout carbohydrate and glycogen replacement. Juices made from fruits are also an excellent choice. The following step is to consume a high-quality protein source. A whey protein drink should do the trick quite well in this situation. As with pre-workout meals, post-workout meals must be consumed promptly. It is recommended to replenish your body's nutritional requirements within 30 minutes of finishing an exercise.

Another nugget of wisdom: On workout days, increase your calorie intake by omitting post-workout meals from your daily calorie count. This assists in ensuring that you consume approximately 25% more calories on workout days. The logic behind this technique is that an intense workout burns many calories, which must be replaced to maintain nutritional balance.

HOW TO STRENGTHEN MUSCLE - YOUR COMPLETE, NONSENSE GUIDE

The most heinous thing you could do when you first begin your muscle-building journey is to attempt to replicate what you see in muscle-building and body-building magazines. Not attempt to replicate the techniques used by professional bodybuilders. You're just getting started, while they're heavily steroid-addicted (which means they can make gains on just about any program, even unhealthy ones).

If you're a common man or woman, you need to take a straightforward approach to build muscle quickly. Additionally, you will require a guide to ensure that you do not overdo it at first (which ultimately harms your progress).

Keep reading to learn more...

How to build muscle - ten quick tips!

Here it is, the one-and-only "no-nonsense" guide you will ever require:

1. Prioritize Strength –

Greater strength always results in increased muscle mass. Additionally, being extremely large and lacking strength is embarrassing. Additionally, strength serves as a foundation for all physical abilities. If you're an athlete looking to improve your endurance, speed, agility, and so on, strengthening your body will help you achieve these goals.

* Body Weight Training - I recommend beginning with body weight (BW) training first, as you should master your body weight before attempting to lift heavier weights, such as iron. Pushups, Pullups, Dips, Squats, Pistols, Crunches, and V-Situps are excellent exercises. When the easier versions of each move become too easy, progress to the more difficult versions. Additionally, BW training is beneficial for tendon strength.

* Resistance Training - Resistance training is excellent for strength development. Additionally, you do not require an abundance of costly equipment. To get started, you'll need an Olympic weightlifting bar set. However, you should always ensure that you are lifting properly. As always, begin with a blank bar and work your way up.

* Kettlebell Training - Kettlebell training is also an excellent way to increase strength. You develop strength at unusual

angles and can perform Olympic-style movements such as the snatch, clean, and jerk with significantly less training than with a barbell. These exercises are relatively simple to master. Additionally, there is less weight to fall on you or the floor if something goes wrong.

2. Utilize Free Weights Whenever Possible –

Avoid weight "machines" at all costs. With a barbell, perform the exercises that will build your strength. Compound exercises such as the squat, deadlift, bench press, and overhead press will greatly impact your strength and physique.

Additional reasons to lift only free weights (specifically, barbells) include the following:

* It's more secure - unlike with machines, you're not performing unnatural, assisted movements. Strength is developed with barbells and free weights in the movements required. Simultaneously, you strengthen all of your stabilizer muscles.

* More Efficient - By engaging more muscles (more stabilizers) when lifting, pressing, and pulling barbells and other free weights, you can build more muscle with less effort.

* More Functional-When you lift heavy objects off the floor... over your head and explosively, perform the same activity as you would in real life. This means that the strength you develop in the gym will carry over into other aspects of your life.

* All-in-One - With just a barbell and weights, you can perform any exercise to build strength and muscle, burn fat, and get in shape. You do not require a large amount of weight training equipment to consume a lot of space (ideal for a home gym).

* Kettlebells are akin to having an entire gym in the palm of your hand - in the form of a couple of small iron balls. Kettlebells require even less space, making them ideal for use in a home gym or while traveling.

3. Always Perform Compound Exercises –

You want to develop strength and muscle across your entire body, so train it as a single unit. The only exception is if you discover you have a muscle imbalance. You must perform isolation exercises to strengthen the weak muscles and stretch the "too tight" muscles (otherwise, injuries will occur). As an illustration

* For the arms, avoid tricep kickbacks and excessive curling; instead, focus on pullups, pushups, presses, and snatches.

* Avoid leg extensions and hamstring curls in favor of squats, kettlebell pistols, and deadlifts for your legs.

* For the chest, avoid flys and pec decks; instead, perform bench presses, overhead presses, and dips, among other exercises.

4. Leg Exercises Squats and Deadlifts are both high-

Intensity exercises that work the entire body. As a result, they assist in musculature development throughout the body. (By exercising your legs, you can build muscle in your chest and arms.) You don't want "chicken legs" and a large upper body. Provide something stable for yourself to stand on—firm legs.

You'll look great if you can squat 1.5 times your body weight (which won't take long!) and deadlift 1.5 times your body weight (or more likely 2 times).

5. Complete Body Workouts are Required –

You must perform complete body workouts. You do not need to perform isolated exercises. Why not maximize your investment? Why not maximize your results in the gym in the shortest period possible? Here are seven reasons why total-body workouts are superior for muscle development and fat loss.

If you participate in any sport, complete body training will help you become more athletic and perform better. Kettlebells are excellent full-body tools since several exercises train the complete body, including snatches, cleans, and presses.

6. Recover as Effortlessly as You Work Out –

The more you overtrain, the slower you will progress. Additionally, the larger your muscles are, the more rest you require. You may genuinely grow 30 pounds of muscle in just four hours of exercise - the secret is recuperation. Muscles always build outside of the gym, not in it. Here are the points to consider:

* Take a break. You do not grow in the gym; simply complete three rigorous exercises each week and exit.

When you're not working out at the gym, take a break. Meditation and relaxation are beneficial because they reduce stress and cortisol levels, which aid in muscular growth and fat loss. Consider the quality of your workouts rather than the quantity when determining how much time you spend in the gym.

* Adequate sleep. While you sleep, your body restores itself. During deep sleep, levels of Growth Hormone and Testosterone are boosted. If possible, get eight hours of restful sleep. However, the quality of sleep is more critical than the quantity. That is fantastic if you can squeeze in a fast 20-minute snooze following your workout.

* Consume Enough. Your body requires food for fuel and recovery. Consume only healthy foods (more on that in a moment).

* Consume Water. I aim for one gallon per day. At each meal, consume at least two glasses. Pure water is necessary for hydration and is beneficial for many additional reasons.

7. Maintain a healthy diet.

You want muscle mass, not fat mass, correct? Consume only healthy foods. Anything contained in a box is DANGEROUS. Simply accept it. Allow yourself one "cheat day" per week to avoid going insane trying to eat clean.

On that day, binge on the foods you're trying to avoid since they're terrible for you; this way, you'll get sick of them and won't want to eat them the rest of the week. It's difficult to achieve perfection, so aim to eat well at least 80% of the time. You will require (in ascending order of importance):

* Lean beef, poultry, eggs, whey protein, and milk are all good sources of protein...

* Fruits and vegetables. Broccoli, tomatoes, and spinach, to name a few...

* Fatty acids. Fish oil, extra virgin olive oil, real butter, and nuts, to name a few...

* Berries. Bananas, apples, oranges, and avocados are just a few examples...

* Carbohydrates Whole grain and brown rice, except post-workout carbohydrates

8. Supplement –

While some argue that supplements are unnecessary, I argue that our food supply is nutritionally deficient. Which medication should you take...

* Whey Protein - aids in protein absorption (more on that in a moment)...

* Fish oil - is the healthiest vitamin available.

* Superfood/green beverage - to obtain the necessary vegetable/green goodness

* Multivitamin - to ensure that you receive all of your vitamins AND minerals

* Enzyme formula - promotes quicker healing and general health

* Creatine - aids in muscle growth and has a slew of additional health advantages.

9. Put a premium on protein.

It is stated that 1 gram of protein per pound of bodyweight is required to create muscle. I've never been able to accomplish it consistently, and while I continue to grow muscle and burn fat, I always prioritize protein (in my mind, a meal without protein is not a meal). Additionally, protein has a greater thermogenic effect than other macronutrients, making it beneficial for fat loss. Here are some protein-rich foods:

* red Meat. Ground round, steaks, venison, buffalo, and Cetera

* Fowl. Breast of chicken, whole chicken, turkey, duck, etc.

* Fish, such as tuna, salmon, and flounder...

* Fresh Eggs. (Yes, including the yolk.) Alternatively, use 80/20, or 80 percent white and 20% yolk.

* Dairy products. Milk, cheese, yogurt, and whey protein are all excellent whey protein sources.

10. Never Give Up –

Do not become frustrated if you do not immediately see results. Maintain a pleasant mental attitude; this is critical. Concentrate on the fundamentals, build strength, and develop in modest increments; you'll have come a long way before you realize it. Subscribe to this site and frequently return for additional assistance.

CHAPTER 4
STRENGTHENING OF THE MUSCLE

The general public sometimes misunderstands muscle strengthening as a practice reserved for serious bodybuilders. Bulky muscles, broad chests, and flexed arms in the Arnold Schwarzenegger style are the pictures that come to mind when the muscular building is discussed. However, the entire concept extends beyond that.

Individuals must recognize that muscle building should be a universal goal. It is something that everyone should commit to because it has the potential to significantly improve one's body, even if one is not a bodybuilder. The anxiety of developing too huge and ugly muscles and the fear of accumulating too much "bulk" or weight should not be taken for granted.

When it comes to muscle strengthening, it's critical to keep in mind that everyone's body composition is unique. This is more pronounced in men than in women. Each individual reacts differently to weight training. With women, a low testosterone level ensures that they will not grow an excessive amount of muscle or become bulky when they commit to a strengthening exercise.

Men may respond to strength training faster, but they may always tailor the outcomes of a strengthening routine to their bodies. A man can always set specific goals for his training regimen, improve his appearance, maximize the program, and build muscle mass.

Muscle strengthening is undoubtedly beneficial to those who devote themselves to it. A successful strengthening routine reduces body fat and enhances lean muscle mass. A body with a higher proportion of lean muscle mass can burn calories more efficiently than a body with a lower lean muscle mass. When muscles are strengthened, the body becomes more toned, resulting in a slimmer, compact appearance.

Strengthening muscles improves the body's balance and coordination, lowering the chance of injury and muscle degradation. Additionally, strengthened muscles increase bone mineral density, allowing the body to accomplish athletic and even daily tasks more easily.

Before beginning a muscle-strengthening exercise, you should acquire approval from your physician. The location of strength training activities is critical to your motivation and convenience. You do not need to invest excessively in garments unless you are entirely devoted to recuperating the value of your purchase.

If you overspend on clothing and appear hesitant to continue your strengthening program, you may discover that you've squandered too much money. It's also critical to consult a personal trainer as a beginner strength trainer to ensure By doing so; you maximize the value of your training.

THE BASICS OF STRENGTH TRAINING - STRENGTH TRAINING WORKOUTS AND BENEFITS

You've probably heard of strength training in the gym or from males who regularly visit the gym for bodybuilding. However, this exercise is not only for males; it is critical for everyone seeking a leaner physique and weight loss. As the name implies, strength training engages in workouts that increase muscle strength and mass. Strength training fundamentals include weightlifting, using weight machines, and performing exercises that utilize your body resistance.

The Advantages You Will Receive

This sort of exercise has numerous benefits, including strengthening your muscles, bones, and tendons and boosting your health and fitness. Additionally, it aids in the prevention of injuries and osteoporosis.

Strength training also aids in weight loss, as it increases your metabolism even after your workout, allowing your body to burn more calories. Additionally, it aids in decreasing your blood pressure and harmful cholesterol levels.

The Activities Involved

Before beginning any workouts, it is critical to visit your physician to determine whether your body is prepared for these exercises. To familiarize yourself with the fundamentals of strength training, below are several workouts that fall under this category.

Upper body exercises such as bench press, pull-ups, dips, triceps extensions, and curls can be performed. Squats, lunges, calf raises, leg extensions, and curls are additional fundamental exercises for lower body strength training. You can also train with free weights, such as dumbbells and barbells, or with the weight machines found in most gyms. Additionally, you can perform activities that use your body weight as resistance, such as push-ups.

These exercises are included in the majority of basic strength training programs. However, they are also included in more specialized programs. Among them are maintenance training and circuit training.

You can also choose the workouts based on the area of the body you wish to strengthen. It is also critical to complete your warm-up exercises before beginning these workouts. Warming up is critical because it helps your muscles prepare for rigorous activity and helps you avoid injuries.

Additional Considerations

To ensure that your routines are as effective as possible, you must consider your diet. In this manner, you may educate your body to respond positively to the physical activity you are participating in. To achieve a balanced effect on your body, it's also a good idea to train your full body rather than just your legs or biceps. Additionally, while performing the exercise, practice good breathing techniques and remember to rest your muscles to allow them to regenerate.

It is necessary to understand strength training fundamentals to reap the benefits to avoid wasting your time and know-how to achieve the best results from your exercises.

EXERCISES THAT STRENGTHEN THE MUSCLES

Muscle strength indicates good health and stamina, endurance, resistance, and, of course, strength. When your muscles are toned and strong, you can accomplish a great deal in a short period. Additionally, you are more productive and capable of accomplishing more than someone with untoned muscles.

You may be wondering how these individuals with well-built bodies obtained them and if you, too, can achieve similar physiques. You could be thinking about what type of activities you should engage in. to achieve those toned muscles. Some will cost you money, but if you are truly committed to getting in shape and strengthening your muscles, you may want to take a small risk and invest in some necessary machines.

Exercises for muscle strengthening and toning can be performed with machines, free weights, and equipment that aid in body weight-bearing activities.

The abdominal bench and rowing machine are two machines that assist you tone and building your muscles. The abdominal bench is an excellent way to tone your core muscles. This encompasses the muscles of the upper and lower abdomen and the obliques. On the other side, the rowing machine strengthens your back. It works every muscle in your back and oblique, posterior, chest, and arm muscles. Additionally, it provides excellent cardiovascular exercise.

The free weights can be utilized to perform forearm training. Simply hold the bars parallel to your body and twist your wrists upward and downward. The bench press machine is another type of free weight that you can utilize. The bench press machine is mostly used to tone the pectoral muscles. Additionally, this machine benefits the triceps, anterior deltoids, and serratus anterior.

Simple sit-ups and push-ups can be performed at home without purchasing equipment. Sit-ups assist tone your abdominal muscles. While your feet are linked to a fixed item and your hands are behind your head or crossed at the chest, you need to lift your upper body vertically by bending at the waist. On the other hand, push-ups work the chest, triceps, and shoulders. If the traditional push-up is too difficult for you, begin with your knees on the floor.

Each of these exercises will have a unique effect on your muscles. Each is meant to tone and build specific muscle groups. Once you've determined which muscles are toned by a certain piece of equipment or exercise, you should be able to choose the appropriate workout for muscle strengthening.

CAN YOU STRENGTHEN AND TONE WITHOUT A GYM?

Is a gym or a personal trainer really necessary to get that chiseled, buff body complete with washboard abs, sculpted muscles, and a firm gluteus maximus, affectionately referred to as the rear-end or derriere?

Contrary to popular belief, you do not need to join a gym. to begin your fitness journey. I CONDUCTED EXTENSIVE RESEARCH. I CONDUCTED EXTENSIVE RESEARCH. When I decided to get "in shape," I conducted extensive research. I read articles, conversed with fitness enthusiasts, and downloaded numerous apps to my phone. These supplied critical literature on exercise programs that may be performed using only your weight rather than an ergonomic gym machine.

There are several variables to examine in this case. Your physique serves as the personal template for your work. If anyone should comprehend your body weight, mass, and habits, it should be you.

Rather than attempting to meet the aims or expectations of others, use your potential as a beginning point.

Avoid idealizing a particular cooker-cutter model or a one-size-fits-all philosophy.

Establish short-term goals and create a checklist to track your progress as you reach each milestone.

I'm not opposed to gyms or personal trainers because many individuals, quite simply, require that extra push or incentive to achieve. When we interact with people and share our stories, we create a common dynamic in which we may encourage, uplift, and motivate one another along the way.

However, what about individuals with a busy schedule or who prefer to exercise in the privacy of their own homes? Several viable options can be equally beneficial.

If you live near a park or parkway, this is an excellent resource for aerobic exercises such as running, jumping rope, biking, or even strolling. Cardiovascular exercises are critical because they increase the heart rate, which results in increased blood circulation and oxygen to the cells throughout the body. We require oxygen for respiration, which generates energy and uses lipids and glucose. In a nutshell, we metabolize sugars and fats!

Strengthening and toning should play a significant role, depending on your fitness objective. When we apply force to our muscles, the muscle fibers stretch and tear. The repair and renewal of these fibers cause these tissues to expand and muscle mass to rise. This results in the ability to perform additional exercises due to the restored vitality and vigor of the muscular tissues.

How I strengthened and toned.

When you decide to go on a fitness journey, several factors to consider. It is critical to consider all variables. It is the confluence of critical aspects such as diet, rest, and exercise that will assist you in achieving your fitness objective, as these all work in unison to provide the desired result. I'll briefly review some of the exercise activities that contributed significantly to my physical transformation in this article.

Two devices proved important in my training since they added diversity and provided a simple way to challenge myself. One of these is the resistance band, which can be used for bicep curls, squats, chest presses, shoulder presses, triceps extensions, and calf raises. They are convenient to store;

The workout ball is the other tool. Yes, the large ball resembling a beach ball can be squishy if not properly inflated and force you to reread the description after doubting whether it was a toy or workout equipment.

I Used the Following Supplements.

-I supplemented with multivitamins, which are necessary for proper bodily function. Vitamins are naturally occurring compounds in food, but how many of us have an l-balanced diet that contains all of the key nutrients properly? properly

-Creatine Monohydrate - Creatine is an amino acid-based substance synthesized in the body (building blocks of proteins). It resulted in a rise in the creation of ATP (the cell's energy storage currency), which provided me with more energy and boosted my performance and muscle mass.

****Drink Water - Maintain proper hydration. Sweating results in the loss of water. They are consuming water assists in replenishing this fluid loss. Other electrolyte-containing beverages (such as Gatorade) can also assist replace electrolyte loss, but my love-hate relationship with Gatorade is a story for another day.

A selection of my exercises

I employed circuit training, which is a technique that involves rapidly switching between exercises with little or no rest in between sets. I performed a mixture of the following exercises in three sets of 12 reps at other times. (A rep is an abbreviation for repetition, the number of times an exercise is performed, whereas a set is a sequence of repetitions.) I normally rest between sets for 30-60 seconds before moving on to the next exercise.

Cardio - Among the cardiovascular activities that I performed with vigor and enthusiasm were jumping jacks, jump-roping, and jogging for approximately 5 minutes.

Push-ups - This was my most difficult exercise. I couldn't perform a single push-up when I first started, even if my life relied on it. I'm thrilled to report that I've progressed from "girly" push-ups on my knees to the hardcore military-style push-ups that the drill sergeant screams down recruits' ears. Push-ups are a total-body workout that strengthens the triceps, core, and abdominals.

The best advice I've received about push-ups is to do as many as possible. If you're just capable of completing sets of one rep, that's fine.

Curls of the Biceps - Excellent for obtaining those "weapons" that should serve as a motivator for everyone to exercise. Consider Michelle Obama's toned arms as an example. Do I need to say more?

Planks - An excellent approach to varying your abdominal exercises. Do you recall a few years back when Facebook was swamped with photographs of people planking humorously and amusingly? Planks are genuinely beneficial exercises that involve holding a fixed position for an extended time.

Lunges - These exercises for the lower body target the quadriceps, gluteals, and legs.

Crunches - Who doesn't desire rock-solid, washboard abs? They are unquestionably possible. I primarily used the gym ball for this activity because it provided much-needed support and padding for my back.

Squats - Let's discuss your bootylicious physique—a Brazilian butt-lift without the expense, discomfort, or knife. Additionally, squats improve the leg muscles (quadriceps, hamstrings, and calves), necessary for stability.

Dips - This exercise is beneficial for strengthening the triceps muscles. At home, you can perform triceps dips on a couch or chair.

Several Popular Health/Fitness Myths

Perhaps the most pernicious fallacy I've encountered is that you should drink eight glasses of water daily. Where are the scientific studies and specific findings that substantiate this theoretical nonsense? You must consume water by your body's requirements.

Someone active, such as a construction worker working in direct sunshine, may require more than eight glasses. On the other side, a person who spends most of their time inactive may not require as much alcohol. Of course, there are additional variables to consider, such as age, weight, and health-related issues.

Another prevalent myth is that your toned muscles will deteriorate and convert to fat if you do not adhere to your fitness plan. Erroneous! Muscle and fat are biologically distinct structures, and when you do not exercise, there is no conversion from one to the other. Absence of exercise results in "muscle atrophy," a decrease of muscle mass that makes muscles appear less solid and toned. This effect is not due to conversion to fat.

My point here is that you can accomplish a great deal by working out independently. Using easy exercises, I gradually shaped and defined specific regions of my physique. Making excuses for being unable to attend the gym is neither appropriate nor persuasive. You are the first step toward a toned and healthy body.

Follow your body's natural rhythms and begin your challenges gradually, without attempting to accomplish too much at once. When embarking on any quest or journey, rely on your creative energies and individuality. You do not need to be enslaved. Concepts such as "you must do this" or "do it this way" because these concepts restrict your originality, stifle your creativity, and do not sit well with non-conformists such as yourself.

CHAPTER 5
LEAN AND FIT PILATES

Pilates evolved as a result of Joseph Pilates's diligence and intelligence. Joseph Pilates was born in 1880 in Germany. He suffered from rickets and asthma as a child. He was never particularly athletic, and as a result of his early handicaps, he became committed to assisting others in overcoming theirs. He assisted veterans both during and after World War I., assisting them in regaining their health.

He began experimenting with springs as a technique of resistance for exercising the patient's muscles at this time. He and his wife Clara founded the first Pilates studio in New York City. Joseph Pilates died in 1967, yet his techniques continue to be passed on through his disciples.

Pilates is primarily a resistance training regimen that focuses on stretching and strengthening muscles throughout the body. While some of the concepts in Pilates originated in various types of Yoga, the way they are incorporated into the Pilates approach is unique. Dancers frequently use pilates to strengthen and tone their muscles. Athletes of all types have benefited from these strategies to recover from injuries.

While Pilates has multiple documented benefits for everyone, others criticize the technique. One is that Pilates is not a stand-alone fitness regimen. It omits beneficial cardiovascular exercise. Additionally, if you're aiming to bulk up, Pilates is probably not for you.

Due to the system's lack of emphasis on high-intensity muscular training, the muscle mass gained through Pilates is typically less than that gained through other exercise regimens. However, it has been demonstrated to increase your flexibility and benefit your complete body.

Today, the Pilates approach is available in a variety of forms. Some people were personally taught by Joseph Pilates and have passed on their knowledge to their students in the precise manner they acquired it from the master.

There are other others who have modified the approach or added new exercises yet continue to call it Pilates. Advertising can be deceiving, so make certain that you are getting what you paid for with a professional, licensed instructor.

Whether you are injured or crippled, a beginner or an experienced exerciser, Pilates has a version. After all, it is your body, and you should be able to influence how it is trained.

PILATES' SIX PRINCIPLES

Joseph Pilates, the founder of the Pilates training method, was born as a thin, sickly child in Germany. This frail boy developed into a bodybuilder, professional boxer, and founder of one of the most well-known physical training programs.

Joe Pilates established a system of movements based on yoga, gymnastics, and kung fu that highlighted the significance of breath control and core muscular development.

Pilates originally referred to his physical routine as "Contrology" and discussed it in his now-famous 1945 book "Return to Life Through Contrology." The Pilates method subsequently adopted its founder's name. Joseph Pilates instructed a sizable number of pupils. They continued his work, including Romana Kryzanowska, one of the most renowned Pilates disciples.

In the early 1980s, two of Roman's students, Philip Friedman and Gail Eisen, published a book titled The Pilates Method of Physical and Mental Conditioning. They outlined the six core Pilates principles of concentration, control, center, flow, accuracy, and breathing.

Concentration: Pilates positions are tough for the faint of heart. They frequently require two distinct muscles to perform two distinct tasks concurrently. This necessitates an extremely high level of concentration. And focus. It is currently considered that when mental attention is paired with physical activity, brain functions such as memory and problem solving can improve.

Control: Pilates motions demand complete control of the entire body at all times, hence the term "Contrology" in its original form. Each movement and stance is meticulously studied and rehearsed, ensuring no unnecessary motions or breaths.

According to the Pilates method, all movement originates in the body's center, or core, which comprises the abdomen, lower and upper back, hips, buttocks, and inner thighs. Each Pilates action is fueled by energy that originates in the core and then spreads to the limbs.

Flow: Pilates motions enhance energy efficiency by flowing from one to the next.

Precision: Each movement in the Pilates method must be executed precisely. There is a strong emphasis on form, with the concept that doing one movement flawlessly is more effective than performing numerous poor moves. This concept of excellence in all actions is anticipated to become ingrained in the subconscious mind and permeate all facets of life.

Breathing: Because Pilates places such a premium on proper breathing, it should probably be listed as the first principle. Pilates recognized that increasing oxygen intake and blood circulation could help practically any physical condition. Proper breathing in Pilates entails vigorously exhaling to inhale more thoroughly.

As successive generations of Pilates practitioners have strived to perfect Joe Pilates' program, the method has surely evolved slightly. However, the essential concepts of Pilates remain unchanged, with subsequent generations benefiting from this time-tested approach to physical and mental conditioning.

PILATES CIRCLE - FOR STRENGTH AND FLEXIBILITY

One wish that all humans have is the desire for good health. Having a single workout is unavoidable. No, there is no gain without pain! The concept of fitness has existed for eons. The majority of experts and nonprofessionals believe that you must endure some discomfort to improve.

This is not entirely accurate. The genuine outcomes are only revealed if you are willing to make an effort. You can work out regularly if you discover a way to love it. In today's environment, the Pilates exercise regimen is increasing popularity. It is mostly composed of resistance movements designed to stretch and strengthen muscles throughout the body.

Today, the Pilates approach is available in numerous versions. Joseph Pilates himself invented the Pilate Circle. It was made of a different substance back then than it is now. The quality of the Pilate circle remains the same in terms of core strength, flexibility, and balance. It is adaptable and portable.

Pilate circles, alternatively referred to as exercise rings, magic rings, fitness circles, and various other terms are circular training equipment. They are made of metal or rubber that is malleable. They have a diameter of approximately 13 inches. Typically, they feature cushions on either side for pressing the circle in or out.

It is used in exercising to provide gentle to moderate resistance. It is not meant to present a significant resistance obstacle. If you are a stronger individual seeking a greater muscular challenge, you will not want rubber or even one of the new "light" metals; they squish far too quickly.

The Pilate circles are ideal traveling companions. They lie flat and have a little volume relative to their size. Consider the rubber or "light" version if you are a frequent traveler. If you're looking for something durable, a lot of use in the studio, the standard metal one is excellent. Even with considerable resistance, the standard metal circle is adequate.

Initially, the pads were located on the circle's periphery. Pads on the interior of the circle are also a new trend. The pads on the interior contribute to the Pilate circle's adaptability.

While in a Pilate circle, it is simple to be deceived. These devices are available in a range of configurations. Of brands. Some are very mushy and flimsy. To avoid this, speak with your Pilate instructor and inquire about the brand used in your facility. Purchase one in-store or online from a trusted source. Prices range from $ 20 to $ 75, so they are not prohibitively expensive.

Whether you are injured or incapacitated, a beginner or an experienced exerciser, these Pilate circles are for you; just make sure you have the necessary information and a professional instructor with whom you feel comfortable working.

STRENGTHENING OF THE CENTRAL MUSCLE

Core muscle training is critical for grace, stability, healthy posture, and aging. Your body's core muscles are found in your back and abdominals; imagine a corset composed entirely of muscles beneath your skin. A weakened core can contribute to poor posture., a painful back and neck, and an increased risk of injury. There are a plethora of core strengthening exercises available to everybody, and the greatest ones rely heavily on your body weight.

Strengthening the core muscles is critical for weightlifters, particularly heavier weightlifters. This is because weightlifting primarily targets specific muscle areas, e.g., the bench press primarily targets the chest and pectoral muscles. If you do press-ups on the floor instead of a bench, you will notice that you must also engage your core by contracting your abdominal muscles to maintain your body upright.

As a result, while many weightlifters are satisfied with their results, their core muscles are not receiving the same amount of training, resulting in an imbalance between the core muscles and the other muscle groups. As a result, the body's metabolic rate may increase. Prone to damage.

If you have huge biceps but have never worked on your core, this may explain why You become aware of a twinge in your back. or even pull a muscle when attempting to move a big suitcase, TV, or box. This is why the core muscles are critical, and all training regimens must include some core-strengthening activities.

Any workout in which you must maneuver your body weight demands you to use your core muscles to transfer and stabilize your weight. Have you ever wondered how dancers maintain such excellent posture and stability when performing handstands, twists, and jumps? This is because practically every action performed in dance requires the utilization of the entire body and all of the core muscles.

Hopefully, you now understand why coming to the gym and focusing exclusively on weight machines is not useful to your body's core or strength training. Additionally, you may understand why free weights are considered superior to weight machines. They require you to engage the stability muscles in the weightlifting muscle region.

EXERCISES FOR CORE STRENGTHENING - THE BENEFITS

Historically, most core strengthening exercises were performed by women and taught through "feminine" fitness disciplines such as Pilates, Yoga, dancing, and cheering. However, current research has substantiated the fields' statements regarding the multiple benefits of core strength. As a result, it has expanded throughout the fitness and exercise world and is now regarded as a fundamental component of any regimen to improve general physical health and strength.

This article aims to shed light on the numerous benefits of having a strong core.

1. Prevents and alleviates back pain. Apart from being a technique for achieving fitness, core exercises are effective as a type of rehabilitation, particularly in the case of back discomfort or injury. This is because deconditioned individuals frequently feel lower back pain. This soreness and potential injury are caused by a lack of strength in the

hip flexors, hamstrings, abdominals, and back muscles. Core strengthening exercises develop and support the muscles above, alleviating back discomfort.

2. Decreases the risk of injury. You are more stable and less prone to injury when you have strong core muscles. The weakening or unstable muscles cause numerous illnesses; therefore, you can ward off those potential injuries by engaging in activities that strengthen your core.

Numerous studies have established that core stability is critical for injury prevention among athletes and gym buffs, and various jobs. For example, research has shown that improving flexibility and strength in the trunk and core muscles group resulted in a 42 percent reduction in injuries and a 62 percent reduction in missed work time due to injury over 12 months.

3. Maintains Your Balance. Each year, numerous accidents involving falling occur, which has become the main cause of accidental deaths among individuals over 65. Numerous unfortunate occurrences are the result of improper balance and posture. Improving your core strength can help you avoid this, as your core muscles are responsible for maintaining a steady center of gravity. Additionally, the workouts strengthen the individual muscles and improve their coordination, allowing them to work more efficiently together.

4. Encourages proper posture. In addition to improving balance, core exercise strengthens the erector spine and pelvic region muscles. A solid pelvis will automatically maintain its neutral and straight position, as will your back.

5. Strengthens Your Body. The majority of your extremities or peripheral muscles, such as your arms and legs, rely on your core for additional strength and energy to complete the duties we assign them. Ultimately, a strong core

increases overall physical performance, as demonstrated by ordinary daily activities.

The benefits listed above are just a sampling of the benefits associated with core strengthening activities. Additionally, you should not overlook the aesthetically pleasant reward of a tight pack of abs if you perform them.

CORE TRAINING - SELECTING EXERCISES BASED ON STABILITY

As the science of sports performance training advances, workouts become increasingly effective in translating their effects to daily activities. Exercise scientists and imaginative trainers are constantly developing new and improved methods for assisting people in doing better in their sports and everyday human activities.

Core training is one crucial area that continues to grow rapidly. While this is frequently referred to as abdominal (or 'abs') training, it involves every muscle in your lower torso. Additionally, this region is associated with the health and performance of all of the hip and shoulder muscles.

To put it bluntly, this is the most critical component of any workout. And the workouts you choose make a huge impact on the benefits you get from your total training.

Those who have not yet converted to a stability-focused core training regimen and are still relying on crunches and sit-ups as the cornerstone of their program consider this a plea to make the necessary changes.

What qualifies as a core stability exercise? This straightforward guide can help you determine whether an exercise provides stabilization benefits or not.

When completing any exercise, pay close attention to how your shoulders and hips are positioned. Whatever the drill, if you can maintain a straight line from your shoulder to the same-side hip while your core is engaged, this is a stability exercise.

To be sure, this is a significant simplification. However, this explains why activities such as crunches, sit-ups, side bend with dumbbells, and twists have little effect on abdominal stabilization. The crunch positions the shoulders ahead of the hips, the side bend positions them to the left or right, and the often performed twist rotates either the shoulders or the hips, but not both.

These exercises deviate from the normal movement patterns used by healthy individuals in sports and daily activities. Your body can generate the most force when your midsection is perfectly aligned hip-to-shoulder in every movement possible. Any departure depletes vital power in sports and puts you at a greater risk of injury.

The bridge and side bridge are two excellent examples of simple stability-based exercises (also known as the plank and side plank). They both maintain a straight line from the hip to the shoulder while utilizing gravity to place significant stress on the core muscles when performed correctly.

This strengthens the big abdominal muscles and forces the smaller stabilizers closer to the spine to activate and perform their function. These little fellas are critical for proper posture and other basic activities, yet they are completely ignored in drills without a stabilizing component.

These are just two simple examples of core stability exercises, but countless others provide strong advantages. Improved core stability benefits the complete body's health and function, boosting speed, strength, and power. Consider the improvements in your general health and athletic performance that will eliminate all workouts that do not provide this great combination of advantages and adopt a stability-based approach.

TRAINING THE CORE FOR IMPROVED BODY FUNCTIONS

Core training is the newest exercise trend in the world of fitness. It is dissimilar to exercising for great abs or a six or eight pack. Not everyone understands the underlying fundamentals of rigorous exercise, which has resulted in a great deal of misinformation about this type of exercise.

Everybody wants to have a flawless set of abs to flaunt, but often in the pursuit of ideal abs, we overlook the back discomfort and other physical issues that come with age. This is where core training differentiates itself from simple exercise. The fundamental goal of core training is to promote a more balanced and realistic attitude to health. The primary objective is to enhance both your personality and basic muscle functions.

It is a myth that strenuous exercise targets the lower back muscles primarily. The scope of this type of exercise is significantly broader. Most individuals are ignorant of the full range of functions and advantages associated with this exercise.

On the other hand, Abs training focuses exclusively on the rectus abdominal muscles, oblivious to the transverse abdominal muscles beneath them. Core training focuses on the strengthening of these muscles. One of these types of workout components is strengthening the transverse abdominal muscles.

There are numerous ways this form of workout varies from conventional training. Other types of training are ineffective at strengthening the hips, pelvis, and torso. The workouts are primarily push-pull in nature, aiming toward a one-dimensional physique.

The primary goal of other training programs is to increase the strength of the superficial muscles. This unique workout targets the entire torso, specifically the muscles in the pelvic region. Additionally, this exercise targets the shoulders, hips, and trunk muscles. This provides these muscles with stability and strength. Core training aims to increase the strength and power of the muscles.

For a comprehensive workout, it's critical to concentrate on both movements and all of your body components. Core training focuses on strengthening the body's muscles. Core training serves to increase muscle function and the motions performed by these muscles, which in turn helps to improve overall body function.

THE MOST EFFECTIVE CORE EXERCISES FOR STRENGTH AND STABILITY

Does the following ring a bell? Monday is dedicated to biceps strength. Regardless of the day of the week, you always end your exercises the same way—crunching your way through a dreaded (and very dull) abdominal routine. Are all of these crunches strengthening the muscles in your core? Furthermore, what is the difference between abdominal and core muscles?

First, it's critical to understand that "ab muscles" and "core muscles" do not always refer to the same anatomical area. Rather than that, core muscles include the upper and lower torso (including the abdominals) and the hip, spine, and lower back. Several of these muscles are barely visible on the surface.

However, simply because they are not visible does not mean they are unimportant. Indeed, we use our core muscles every time we sit up, stand, lift something or exercise. Additionally, they safeguard our internal organs and aid our general athletic abilities. Our core muscles stabilize our trunk, allowing our limbs to catch footballs, sprint to the finish line, and make accurate free throws.

"But I'm not an athlete!" you may object. Alternatively, "Why is a core strengthening critical?" A stronger core makes every workout easier, alleviates tension on the other muscles you use to compensate for a weak core (which can wreak havoc on your body alignment and cause other problems), and maintains proper alignment of your upper back muscles. A strong core helps prevent injury and keeps you pounding the pavement, lifting weights at the gym, or swimming that tenth lap, as the case may be.

Elbows and toes planks, side planks, medicine ball chops, stability ball crunches, and jackknives. Core strength exercises should be incorporated throughout your workout and performed with functional aids (such as stability balls and wobble boards) to be most effective over time.

The following are the top five fundamental movements:

1) Planks with elbows and toes: The plank exercise increases endurance and improves the abdominals, back, and other stabilizing muscles. Simply lie on a comfy mat and support your body with your forearms while stretching and resting on your toes.

Elevate your torso off the mat and attempt to create a flat, tabletop surface from head to toe. Your weight should be supported solely by your forearms and toes. Do not allow your stomach to sink inward. Maintain the position for 20–60 seconds and do at least three sets.

2) Side planks: This is an elbows and toes plank variation. On a comfortable mat, lie on your side. As you stack outstretched feet on top of one another and thrust your hips aloft, support your weight on one forearm. Extend your arm straight out to enhance the difficulty. Maintain for 20–60 seconds. Rep at least three times.

3) Medicine ball chops: Position your feet shoulder-width apart and grab a 5-12 pound medicine ball. Raise your arms with both hands on the medical ball. Overhead to your right. This is the initial state. Rotate your trunk as you bring the medicine ball down towards your left foot in a "chopping wood" motion. Bear in mind that your feet remain facing forward. Repeat this motion 10-15 times on each side before switching to the opposite side. Perform at least three sets.

4) Crunches with stability balls: Stability balls can help you improve your balance, flexibility, and torso strength. To perform crunches on a stability ball, comfortably place the ball beneath your lower back. In front of you, cross your arms. or fold them across your chest. When crunching up, avoid pulling your head forward.

Exhale while you concentrate on "pushing" your rib cage down towards your toes and pulling your torso away from the ball—this is the crunch. Maintain this crunch for two beats while maintaining the ball as still as possible as you inhale, gradually lower yourself. Carry out 1-3 sets of 15-20 repetitions.

5) Jack knives: These are difficult core workouts requiring strength and balance. Begin lying on your back, arms extended overhead. Exhale as you maintain straight legs

and arms and elevate your body into a V-position. Maintain balance here for one beat before lowering to the starting position. Rep 8-10 times for a total of at least three sets.

TIPS FOR STRENGTHENING YOUR CORE MUSCLES

Core training has grown in popularity as a fitness philosophy due to its effectiveness in establishing a solid foundation. Here are ten tips for core exercise.

Tip #1: Make Your Abdominal Muscles Active

Abdominal muscles are critical for core stability. Before the arms and legs can move, the deep abdominal muscles contract to stabilize the spine. The drawing-in movement and the plank are excellent abdominal muscle activation workouts.

Tip #2: Strengthen the Muscles in Your Lower Back

Lower back muscles are frequently overlooked in exercise programs, most likely due to vanity. I've never heard someone ask, "Do you know any decent lower back exercises?" Many people in fitness are so focused on achieving six-pack abs and a flat stomach that they overlook their back.

Back muscles are equally as vital as stomach muscles. To possess a robust core, you must have strong abdominal and back muscles.

Tip #3: Develop an Ability to Engage the Pelvic Floor

Although the Pelvic Floor muscles receive the most attention when discussing sexual dysfunction or bladder control issues, they are critical for pelvic and lumbar spine stabilization. They do work the stomach and back muscles. You must contract the pelvic floor muscles as if you were preventing yourself from going to the bathroom to engage them.

#4: Perform Balance Exercises

Balance Exercises are performed on one leg or an unstable surface. Your center of gravity alters as you stand on one leg. You require your core muscles to work harder to maintain your alignment. Balance exercises are a critical component of any exercise program.

Tip #5: Strengthen the Scapular and Rotator Cuff Muscles

The term "core" refers to more than just your spine. Your core is comprised of the shoulder and scapular stabilizers. When your scapula is stable, you are less likely to sustain shoulder problems and perform better. Scapular and rotator cuff exercises should be included in your core workout.

Tip #6: Strengthen your Gluteus Maximus

Hip stabilizers are also included in the core. The glutes are attached to the pelvis and are responsible for hip position control. Pelvic and hip stability is compromised when the glutes are weak or inefficient. Bridges are an excellent workout for strengthening the glutes and stabilizing the core.

Tip #7: Prioritize Stabilization and Endurance Training.

Core stabilization exercises involve little to no movement in the spine area. When beginning a core program, it is critical to establish a stable foundation. If you first focus on stability, you will see bigger gains in strength and speed. The plank is an excellent exercise for core stabilization.

Tip #8: Train for Strength Second

Once you have a decent platform of stability, proceed to grow stronger. Strength workouts push your stomach and back muscles over a vast motion range. Excellent strength exercises are crunches on a Swiss Ball and a machine-assisted lower back extension.

Third Tip: Train for Strength and Speed

Once you've established a foundation of stability and strength, you may construct your speed more efficiently. In addition, if you have a firm foundation, you will be less likely to become hurt and your performance will develop more quickly. Power workouts are performed quickly and explosively—exercises involving medicine balls and leaping assist in developing the strength of your core muscles.

Tip #10: Experiment with a Variety of Core Exercise Equipment

Numerous tools can help you improve your core training. Exercise balls, Reebok Core Boards, and Bosu Balls are excellent instruments for improving coordination and balance. When exercising on less stable surfaces, your core muscles have to work considerably harder to maintain your body's stability.

CHAPTER 6
ANTI-AGING AND VIBRATIONAL FITNESS

What is vibrational fitness, and how does it work? Vibrational fitness (full body vibration) is an exercise that requires you to perform activities on a vibrating platform. These vibrations induce your muscles to contract automatically and independently of your will. How does this relate to anti-aging?

I'm glad you inquired. Seniors are more likely to suffer from falls, osteoporosis, and hip fractures. This is likely to become a greater worry in the coming years as the baby boomers age. This can put these persons' mobility and independence in danger. Apart from the misery that this might bring the individual and their family, it also increases healthcare costs.

The apparent response is an exercise to build muscles and bones while improving balance and postural stability. You should focus on strength workouts performed in a standing position. After all, if strength and stability are required while standing and walking, you should train while standing to maximize carryover. While standing, you must maintain three-dimensional stability.

However, some seniors may have trouble exercising on their feet due to a lack of mobility and balance, frequently compounded by previous injuries. This is the point at which vibrational fitness enters the picture. It enables those with poor balance and mobility to begin in a partial squat position, if necessary while holding onto handles in front of them. Initially, the exercises do not require the user to move; the vibrations contract the muscles instinctively for them.

Their mechanoreceptors, which detect movement and force, are stimulated, which aids with strength and balance while standing - the most critical posture. Additionally, you can set someone on the platform with one foot, knee slightly bent, to replicate the balance required while walking. They can then bend their knees more for increased strength as they develop accustomed to this.

Over time, these static positions will evolve into dynamic ones, enhancing their capacity to maintain stability when moving, such as rising from a chair or bending over to pick something up off the floor. Activities that may be difficult for some seniors to complete. I propose working on these movements in your 40s and 50s to avoid this trouble in the first place.

Additional strength and mobility training would benefit anyone performing whole-body vibration training. The activation of fast-twitch muscle fibers is one of the benefits of exercising on a vibrating platform. These fibers are critical for overall body strength, and if they are not particularly exercised with some form of resistance, they will lose size and function as you age. This can raise your risk of falling or make climbing stairs more difficult. As a result, they are critical to train.

One of these platforms, the Power-Plate, was proven in one study to boost lower body muscle strength and speed of movement in women aged 58 to 74. Another set of women enhanced their lower body strength by training on typical weight machines. However, only Power-Plate users increased their speed of movement. Rapid muscular contraction may mean the difference between falling and not falling.

HOW DO VIBRATION PLATFORMS IMPROVE MUSCLE AND BONE STRENGTH?

How do vibration platforms work?

Vibration Platforms are fitness devices that have a vibrating or oscillating platform. When you stand, sit on the platform, or perform a workout, mechanical energy oscillations are communicated to your entire body. This is one of the reasons it is sometimes referred to as Whole Body Exercise Vibration Training.

The vibration plate generates extremely quick muscle contractions thirty to fifty times per second, continuously working your muscles. These contractions strengthen muscle and bone density, increase flexibility, burn fat, boost metabolism, improve circulation, and increase cellular oxygen and nutrient supply, all of which help delay the degenerative/aging process! The platform descends by either 2 or 4 millimeters. This is a very delicate little drop.

For example, suppose you are standing on the vibration plate with a slight knee bend. Once the platform is lowered by two millimeters, your muscle is rapidly lengthened or stretched. When this occurs, the body responds by rapidly tightening the muscle. By the time it does so, the platform has already returned to its initial position. The platform drops once again, and the process is repeated.

Due to the platform's design, you may achieve a maximum of 50 muscle contractions each second! You can truly obtain 3000 safe and moderate muscle contractions in one minute. This is comparable to performing 3000 knee bends. Without the platform, you can only imagine how long that would take.

Whatever your physical state, vibration training will cause the subconscious stretch reflexes to tighten practically all of your muscles simultaneously. This compares to conventional training, which utilizes only 46% of muscle fibers.

Traditional training strengthens muscles by causing your body to react to the additional resistance generated by the weights above and beyond normal gravity. Vibration Training causes your body to respond to acceleration rather than additional weight, which is more powerful than conventional training stimuli. And one that is repeated thirty or fifty times every second. Your body must adapt even more to cope with the increased load and thus attain your training goals faster. Additionally, the vibrations stimulate the synthesis of regenerative and repair hormones, enhance blood circulation in the skin and muscles, strengthen bone tissue, promote lymph drainage, and elevate the basal metabolic rate.

All of this results in enhanced strength, speed, stamina, rapid muscle and tissue healing, greater flexibility, mobility, coordination, anti cellulitis, collagen enhancement, and fat loss. The idea of "more is better" does not apply to vibration training. You appear and feel fitter, but you are not required to train more intensely.

The Vibration Plate's added value is enhanced training quality and effectiveness, allowing you to minimize your sessions and recover faster. Due to the vibrating machine's greater muscle activation than conventional training, less time is necessary to engage all muscle groups thoroughly.

A one-minute workout on this vibrating platform increases energy expenditure and strengthens the muscles.

Additionally to these muscular contractions, vibration training can work a broader range of muscles.

Because the vibration action causes muscles to contract involuntarily, all muscles involved in the activity will be stimulated. Indeed, with routine exercise such as weight lifting, just 40% of your muscles will be activated. With vibration exercise, that figure can approach 100%.

You will obtain more muscle contractions in a shorter period, but you will also work more muscles throughout this time. This contributes to vibration training being a safe and effective exercise method. This is accomplished with the least strain on the joints and ligaments.

Static or dynamic actions such as standing, sitting, kneeling, lying, and placing your hands on it are permitted. Almost any exercise can be performed on a vibration platform, from a conventional gym workout to reclining in a chair and resting your feet.

Strength Training Benefits

Force equals mass multiplied by acceleration

Do not be afraid of this formula! This indicates the following: When we exercise our muscles, we utilize force to increase or decrease our lifting capacity. There are two methods to build strength: lifting heavier weights (raising the mass to generate more force) or lifting lighter weights faster (keeping the same weight but increasing the acceleration).

Wave vibration workout focuses on acceleration (fast movement of the platform) rather than weight lifted, putting less strain on your joints and ligaments. Beneficial effects on circulation Gentle, fast contractions enable the muscle to function as a pump, increasing blood flow throughout the circulatory system.

This causes the body to eliminate waste items much more quickly, improving circulation and healing. Beneficial effects on the bone Vibration exercise is beneficial for bone health. This is by Wolffe's law, which stipulates that bone responds to physical stress. Rapid muscular contractions produced by the vibration platform result in enhanced strength and the application of beneficial stresses to the bone.

Advantages for Geriatrics

Aging is not just about adding years to one's life but also about improving one's quality of life. The term 'functional age' is far more significant than 'chronological age.' This is defined as an individual's capacity to retain particular characteristics as they age, such as strength, balance, and agility. Exercise has been demonstrated to be advantageous. In numerous studies. In resolving several of these issues.

Inactivity and Aging

After 40, muscle loss happens at 1% every year. Muscle strength is inversely proportional to bone density. Muscle mass and strength loss can affect bone density. Muscle weakness may raise the risk of falls and fractures. Exercise programs for the elderly must be safe, moderate, and effective. Whole-body vibration has gained popularity as a kind of exercise to combat the consequences of inactivity and aging. A recent study has demonstrated good outcomes. These findings have sparked more research worldwide, reiterating the importance of vibration exercise in promoting good aging.

Vibration Exercise and Aging

Increased performance on the chair rising test, indicating increased muscle strength

Reduced risk of falling and an increase in health-related quality of life

Capacity to increase ambulatory competence (walking ability) in older women

Beneficial for balance and movement among residents of nursing homes who have a low level of functional reliance

Vibration exercise has a high rate of compliance.

The scientific ideas that underpin vibration training are as follows:

The reflex of Myotatic Stretch

The reflex of Tonic Vibration

Exercise-Induced Neurological Adaptation The GTO is energized (Golgi Tendon Organ)

Recruitment of Motor Units at the Optimal Level

Increased acceleration results in increased force and power output. Effects of the Stretch-Shortening-Cycle (SSC) Model on the Hormonal System

Circulatory System Effects

The effect on the skeletal system is due to the adaption of Wolff's Law, which shifts the force/velocity curve to the right (faster strength gains)

Exercise is a good means of preventing impairment linked with osteoporosis progression. Exercises including weight-bearing and resistance training are frequently recommended. However, traditional rigorous exercise programs have a low long-term compliance rate and may increase fracture risk.

Whole-body vibration exercise can be viewed as a good substitute for or addition to traditional training. It enables an individual to get comparable outcomes to conventional training in a fraction of the time, enhancing compliance. Mechanical tension generated by muscle contractions is critical for bone strength maintenance. Vibration exercises may be a useful technique for reducing the start and progression of osteoporosis due to their capacity to increase muscle force and power.

Whole-body vibration has been shown to improve blood flow. Gentle, fast contractions are repeated at a high rate causing the muscle to behave as a pump, increasing blood flow throughout the peripheral circulatory system. This leads to the body eliminating waste items much more quickly, which aids in healing.

Summary of the consequences of vibration exercise:

Three months of vibration exercise (maximum time 20 minutes) results in incomparable strength increase to one hour of conventional strength training.

After vibration training, blood circulation is doubled, resulting in the body eliminating waste materials much more quickly, boosting recovery.

Vibration training of varying duration boosts force and power output.

Training has a significant physiological effect (increasing testosterone and growth hormone while decreasing cortisol, the stress hormone'). Enhanced adaptability Enhancement of explosive force

Increases in explosive strength from ten minutes of vibration training each day for ten days are comparable to those obtained from 200 drop-jumps from 24 inches twice a week for a year.

Accelerated improvements in neural adaptation, resulting in a shift to the right on the force/velocity curve (faster strength gains)

FOR OLDER ADULTS, WHOLE-BODY VIBRATION EXERCISE AND VIBRATION TRAINING PREVENT FALLS

With an aging population, balance and stability issues and falls resulting in catastrophic damage are becoming a serious concern that requires a universal solution. Each year, 33% of adults aged 65 and above fall and get an injury. These falls have become a severe issue for this age group, as they are the primary cause of death. 40% of these catastrophic injury falls result in shattered or fractured hips, and 50% result in permanent impairment, with the patient never regaining full functional ability.

As we age, our muscles deteriorate and our bones deteriorate. Density and become brittle, and our balance and coordination deteriorate significantly. As these difficulties worsen, a compounding effect occurs. The weaker someone grows, the less active they become; the less active an individual becomes, the more rapidly these difficulties escalate, resulting in more inactivity. This compounding effect results in a dramatic increase in the number of falls and the injuries due to them.

Physical conditions such as weakened muscles, low stamina, impaired reflexes and coordination, and decreased bone strength all significantly impact the chance of falling. Regrettably, it is more usual for individuals suffering from these side effects to be prescribed prescription drugs than to be placed on a fitness program. According to research, prescription medicines have been linked directly to increased falls in these adults. (As depicted in Figure 1 below)

According to studies, 20% of men and women aged 65 and over were unaware of the cause of their falls, preventing them from getting preventative therapy. Over 43 million Americans, most of whom are female, are affected by osteoporosis (68 percent). This age group needs to receive preventative therapy to maintain an active, safe, and healthy lifestyle.

A Better Way - Drug-Free Treatment

Given that research indicates that prescription medications are not the optimal solution to this problem, what is the alternative?

While whole-body vibration training has existed for decades, it has only lately made its way to North America, where it is being employed by physicians, therapists, and trainers. Hundreds of research studies have been conducted on the technology over the last 15 years to prevent bone loss, build muscle, improve balance and agility, raise beneficial hormones and metabolism, and aid in weight loss, to mention a few. Numerous physicians have embraced the technology as a safe and effective alternative to

To begin, let us define whole-body vibration and its mechanism of action.

The Mechanisms of Whole-Body Vibration Training and Vibration Exercise

There are two unique varieties available on the market of WBV platforms, each of which operates differently and exhibits distinct characteristics:

Triangular in shape, Oscillating vibration platforms oscillate vertically and horizontally in a see-saw pattern between 1 and 10 millimeters. The most prevalent type

2. Tri-planar platforms shake only 1 to 4mm vertically and horizontally. Additional training for sports

Vibration exercise devices induce the "stretch reflex," or involuntary muscular contractions. The tendon is stretched and then involuntarily contracted as the platform descends. The movement is repeated as the platform returns to its initial position. This occurs very rapidly, up to 30 times per second or 30Hz, eliciting 35 muscle spasms per second. The vibration frequency ranges from 5 to 30Hz, and the workout lasts up to 20 minutes.

Vibration Exercise Training is a form of resistance training that does not require weights and does not place as much strain on the joints as conventional exercise training does. Instead of "heavyweights" and the stress associated with them, force is applied by "acceleration."

Strength and Balance Have an Effect

Strength and balance are inextricably linked, so older adults who are weaker are more prone to falling. According to research, knee strength alone accounts for 40% of a person's balance and agility. This is a significant factor in the elderly with osteoarthritis.

Research conducted on this group revealed that as strength grew, the likelihood of falling reduced dramatically, implying a strong correlation between lower-body strength, balance, and agility. Even modest gains in muscle strength significantly affect balance and fall.

Vibration Exercise is extremely helpful in activating these muscles and preventing falls in older adults. Vibration Fitness is also beneficial for older adults who have difficulties exercising.

Older Adults' Strength and Power

Strength improvements have been phenomenal with vibration exercise. Studies indicate an 18% increase in the chair rising test for those over 60, which involves standing from a sitting posture solely using your legs.

Falls are frequently the cause of common injuries such as hip fractures. At the same time, exercising consistently is the most effective preventative measure. Many older adults cannot exercise properly to improve muscular strength. Vibration exercise equipment has been demonstrated to efficiently increase muscle strength in older persons, reducing falls and damage.

People often struggle to maintain a fitness regimen due to exhaustion or boredom. According to research, people are significantly more receptive to and committed to whole-body vibration than regular exercise. The primary draws were as follows:

1. Rapid and efficient

2. It is possible to perform it at home (many disliked going to a gym)

3. An energizing workout that leaves you feeling more energized

4. Appreciate the way they feel afterward

5. More pleasurable than more typical forms of exercise

6. Therapeutic, alleviated joint discomfort, and so forth.

7. Extremely safe; I had no concerns about injury.

Whole-body vibration exercise has been demonstrated to improve strength in the same way that traditional resistance training does, particularly in older persons, without the risk of damage associated with resistance training.

A Synopsis of the Research on Vibration Exercise Machines

The following conclusions are drawn from this assessment of the research on Vibration Exercise Machines:

1. Vibration Exercise improves strength, power, and fitness.

2. Vibration Exercise is beneficial for improving balance and agility.

3. Vibration Fitness is an excellent way to increase bone mass.

4. Whole-body vibration exercises can help older persons avoid falls and injuries.

5. Vibration exercise improves balance and postural control, particularly in individuals with low fitness levels.

6. Vibration training appears relatively safe, with few reported adverse effects.

7. Vibration Exercise has a very high rate of usage over time.

THE BIGGEST WORKOUT "MISTAKES" AND HOW TO CORRECT THEM

Quite frequently, the exerciser and even the personal trainer or coach are unaware of these errors, reducing the exercise's effectiveness and putting themselves at risk of injury. This list describes each "mistake" and includes a recommended "correction." This list may prove useful in grading yourself or your trainer.

Ineffective pre-workout warm-up

A warm-purpose-up is to gradually acclimate the body to the increased stress of the upcoming exercise session. A 5- to 10-minute bout of moderate-intensity cycling, treadmill walking, elliptical work, or even sports-specific movements will be sufficient to induce a mild, sustained stretch.

These activities increase blood flow to the muscles (including the heart) and core muscle temperature, resulting in increased joint flexibility and range of motion and possibly a reduction in injury.

Frequently, exercisers take things too far when warming up; they either skip it entirely or "pre-fatigue" by running fast for 15 to 20 minutes (or longer) before their practice. This has the desired effect. Of depleting necessary muscle carbohydrate stores (glycogen) for the upcoming strength training/bodybuilding session.

Suppose the goal of the exercise is to lose weight. It is preferable to perform extended aerobic exercise or interval training following a bout of severe strength exercise, as the body will likely burn more fat for fuel due to the depleted glycogen stores.

Stretching that is ineffective

Many individuals and personal trainers are unaware of how to perform stretches properly. For instance, when performing a static hamstring stretch on the floor with the leg straight up in the air, it is critical to press the opposing leg into the floor to prevent the pelvis from tilting excessively posteriorly (backward). Posterior tilting will reduce the stretch's effectiveness.

When doing a dynamic stretch such as a lunge to extend, the groin and thigh muscle and the spine (and pelvis, must maintain an upright position, and parallel to the floor; otherwise, the stretch is ineffective. Stretching in the standing position while grasping or pressing against an external source of stability deprives the exerciser of the entire benefit.

At the start of the exercise, practicing dynamic stretches with proper technique in unsupported standing and lunge-type poses may be advantageous. This addresses balance (core stability) and flexibility simultaneously as it prepares the body and joints for movement during the subsequent strength training program. Static stretching may be more beneficial near the conclusion of a training session when the muscles are warm and malleable.

Excessive reliance on machinery

As stated in earlier articles on our website, exercise machines exclusively deprive the core muscles of stimulation and push them to work in isolation or static, non-functional patterns. While certain machines, such as leg press machines and aided pull-up/dip machines, have their place, workouts that emphasize the body's intrinsic stability system (core) are superior for improving movement function and also allow for much more creativity and pleasure.

While exercise machines benefit from introducing resistance training and bodybuilding, they should not be used primarily. An excellent recommendation is to strike a balance between exercises that need the body to maintain its equilibrium and balance (free weights, standing/lunging exercises) and typical machine and assisted workouts that allow more muscle development.

Inadequate exercise technique

Ultimately, the quality of the exercise matters most, not the amount. It's all too easy to sacrifice form for function and accomplishes many more repetitions of an exercise with bad technique than with strict biomechanically accurate technique. Thus, it makes sense that the most difficult part of learning and control is proper technique, which is frequently acquired only via experience and trial and error.

A novice exerciser should engage in the services of a qualified and experienced personal trainer to shorten the learning curve and get it right from the start. For instance, a great way to judge the quality of your or your instructor's squat form is to look at the back of the head about the back of the heel. The spine should be straight (not curved), and the back of the head should remain parallel to the back of the heel (flat) throughout the movement.

Throughout the exercise, the barbell should essentially move in a near-vertical line. As the bar advances, it produces increasing stresses on the spine and intervertebral discs, similar to the arm of a crane. Lifting raises the risk of spinal and connective tissue injury, including discs, muscles, and ligaments.

During abdominal workouts, keeping the feet down and throwing the legs

When executing several sit-ups, an exerciser's feet should never be held down or hooked under a bed/door, as this allows the hip flexor (groin) muscles to accomplish the majority of the effort. The lower abdominals stabilize the pelvis during a sit-up by squeezing the low back into the floor. If the abdominals get fatigued or insufficiently strong to keep the low back flat and the feet stable, the hip flexors may cause the pelvis to tilt forward and the development of a "hole" in the lower back.

Sit-ups performed with a forward-tilted pelvis tend to strain the low back and stretch and weaken the abdominal muscles rather than strengthen them. The same issues might arise when both legs are elevated straight into the air and flung toward the floor by a partner. If the lower abdominals cannot maintain a flat pelvis as the legs approach the floor, this exercise will significantly strain the lower back muscles. A more effective alternative to concentrating on the lower abdominals is reverse curls or hanging knee lifts.

Sustaining a firm grip on the front or side rails of a treadmill

This is a frequent occurrence in any gym or fitness facility: a person steps onto a treadmill and gradually increases the speed and slope. As the inclination increases, the individual grasps the front or sidebars for dear life to avoid being hurled from the machine. Because the arms are practically holding the body up, the rail holding effectively negates the benefit of the increased intensity demands provided by the inclination.

Holding the railings also has a detrimental effect on normal walking/running biomechanics; the absence of an arm swing may result in unnecessary tension on muscles and connective tissue, particularly in the pelvis and low back. Additionally, rail holding reduces the core/balance training stimulus required to walk/run unassisted.

Finally, since most individuals use treadmills to undertake aerobic exercise, Why would you want to lose weight? Want to prevent the arms from moving, which contributes to energy expenditure?

Exercise progression that is ineffective

Any exercise session should follow a logical sequence to achieve the best results. Often, exercisers and trainers do not prioritize exercise order, switching from one exercise to another with no apparent sequence. Exercise order is very important to the eventual results and should be motivated by the chosen exercises' neuromuscular and energy system demands. For example, core exercises that require concentration and precise form should be performed effectively. At the same time, the individual is "fresh" - immediately following a brief Warm-up and stretching exercises.

Core conditioning may be followed by strength conditioning. (as appropriate), This exercise also requires the exerciser to be rested and refueled following an effective performance. For example, multiple joint strength training (squats, lunges, bench press, and shoulder press) should follow power training, as these exercises consume a significant amount of energy.

Alternate upper- and lower-body exercises or use the "pull/push" rule: begin with a pulling exercise and end with a pushing exercise. Because most isolated exercises, such as tricep extensions, bicep curls, and sit-ups, take significantly less energy, they can be performed near the session's conclusion.

Attempting to combine stabilization and mobilization exercises

The core muscles stabilize the pelvis in its "neutral" position (as in standing upright with perfect posture). The pelvic muscles such as the hamstrings, big back muscles, and hip flexors are mobilizing muscles; They rotate the pelvis forward and backward and side to side. To allow for physical movement. It is extremely difficult to develop stability and mobility in a single exercise because they are technically opposed motions.

For instance, executing squats (which require pelvic movement) on a BOSU ball or standing on inflatable discs or foam rollers is unlikely to help strengthen the core. Curl-ups on an exercise ball, on the other hand, are unlikely to enhance core strength since they target the muscles that push the pelvis backward.

Static positions such as bridging and standing are ideal for performing core exercises. Thus, it is advantageous to concentrate on stabilizing strength and mobilizing strength separately rather than concurrently. Before working the arms and legs, establish a core stability and flexibility foundation. Leg strength can be increased significantly when the foot is in contact with a firm surface (such as the ground) - after all, this is how we work in daily life.

Exercise progression is incorrect

Exercisers, personal trainers, and coaches frequently struggle to comprehend functional exercise progressions. They watch others completing an exercise and decide to include it in their own or their client's program. However, it is possible that the individual they watched executing the exercise did it in a functional and organized manner. When an exerciser undertakes an exercise for which they are physically untrained, they run the risk of injury and performing the movement incorrectly.

The proverb JUNK IN = JUNK OUT also applies to exercise because the brain recalls and keeps positive and negative motor and movement patterns; the proverb JUNK IN = JUNK OUT also applies to exercise. A helpful approach is to strengthen from the inside out, rather than the outside in, by emphasizing flexibility and stability. These are the necessary conditions for successfully performing functional motions such as squats, lunges, and sport-specific movements.

Thus, static stability and stretching lead to dynamic stability training, leading strength training and power training. Attempting to condition and strengthen the body from the "outside-in" rather than the "inside out" will yield no adequate results. Any workout program should begin by establishing a foundation (core stability, cardiovascular fitness) and gradually "build" on it to increase performance, strength, and function.

In a squat, place blocks beneath the heels.

Placing blocks beneath the heels is typical technique trainers and exercisers use to compensate for tight calf muscles (soleus) or focus on the quads (thigh muscles). Often, exercisers observe others performing squats in this manner and attempt to replicate them. This practice is not recommended since it simply "gives in" to the ankle's lack of flexibility and does not improve the quality of this highly functional movement.

Additionally, raising the heels places the ankle in an unstable, plantarflexed position, increasing its susceptibility to injury - especially a lateral ankle sprain—the body's center of mass moves. From the midfoot to the toes in this position, it increases the probability of a loss of balance and possible injury. Controlling the bar placement on the back is safer to target either the quadriceps or the hamstrings and glutes.

The bar is held in place by the posterior deltoids (shoulder muscles) near the base of the neck in the high position, which effectively targets the quadriceps muscles. When the bar is in a low position, it rests further back, at the level of the middle trapezius, across the posterior deltoid (top of the shoulder blades).This posture results in a greater load being shifted to the hamstring and glute muscles.

OVER- AND UNDER-TRAINING

When it comes to personal fitness, maintaining a healthy balance is critical. How do you know when to ramp up your fitness routine? How can you know if your body is capable of enduring strenuous exercises? Are you training if you are not constantly weary and tired? These questions pertain to determining the precise amount of optimal exercise for your body. It is critical to grasp the difference between excessive and insufficient training.

Training excessively:

Overtraining is a word that refers to pushing your body too hard while exercising. When you exercise consistently, your fitness level will gradually improve. It's worth noting that stressing or straining your muscles is just as critical as adequate rest following exercise to build and strengthen your muscles. Muscle proteins required for development and repair are created exclusively during rest periods following exercise. If you train or exercise excessively, you risk developing consequences such as high blood pressure and sleep problems. Overtraining can also result in injury, resulting in muscular damage.

How do I tell when I've overtrained?

You effectively deny yourself adequate recovery time between workout sessions when you overtrain. This could also suggest that you execute activities at a very high intensity for an extended period. This typically results in a loss in immunity, exposing you to frequent colds and illnesses. Muscles may also cause pain, and minor injuries may occur. All of these factors suggest that you may have been overtrained.

What am I to do?

Allow yourself a rest. Relax and sleep well to allow your body to repair itself.

During training

Undertraining occurs as a result of inactivity over an extended period. Undertraining is the polar opposite of overtraining. The recovery period between workouts is extended beyond what is essential, and the intensity of the workouts is minimal. Undertraining is frequently the result of laziness and a lack of commitment to an exercise plan. Extreme inactivity can result in heart disease, obesity, diabetes, cancer, and even depression.

How am I aware that I am undergoing training?

This is a much more straightforward concept to grasp Than excessive training. You will be aware if you have missed an exercise session. Sleepiness, laziness, and an aversion to any type of work are all indicators of inadequate training.

What am I to do?

The solution is fairly straightforward. It is time for you to begin exercising to maintain your body physically active. Begin by jogging and performing simple stretches in the mornings. Maintain physical activity and avoid becoming a couch potato.

Returning to creating a balance, moderation is critical for physical training. It's comparable to cooking vegetables. If you cook them too quickly, they remain raw, and they lose vital nutrients if you cook them too long. Training is also not dissimilar. Take care not to over-or under-train but to establish the proper balance.

CONCLUSION

Before beginning a muscle-building program, it is critical to understand its purpose. Muscle is simply the tissue in our body that provides us with the necessary power to move in various directions. As bodybuilders, our primary focus is on skeletal muscle. What exercises can we perform to improve our bodies and increase muscle? It is critical to remember that each individual has a unique body mass.

We will be unable to acquire the body we desire if we continue to read Body-building magazines. We must approach the entire process differently. That is a way that is both appropriate and advantageous to us. The technique you should take to muscle gain is staged and detailed in the many procedures to be followed.

Muscles must be exercised to be strengthened. This necessitates weight training. You can begin with modest weights and gradually increase them. The objective is to push oneself outside of one's comfort zone. If you believe you can easily bear certain weight, it's time to increase it.

It is always preferable to grow muscles with a barbell or dumbbell rather than a machine. Free weights are safe to use since they take advantage of the body's natural movements. They are also effective since they demand your balance and control weight, which aids in muscular growth. Additionally, they are useful and adaptable.

These exercises require the simultaneous usage of numerous muscles. This is crucial if you intend to begin muscle growing. Pull-ups and chin-ups need you to bear your weight. They are the best upper body and muscle mass strength training. Barbell rows are another technique that helps strengthen your upper back, lower back, lats, and traps.

The bench press is a very popular bodybuilding technique that assists muscle and strength development. This workout helps you increase strength in your upper body. Additionally, it engages the front shoulder and triceps muscles. The overhead press is another exercise that is beneficial for muscular building. It works out the entire body. Each shoulder head receives an equal amount of labor. Dips are another series of exercises that put your upper body through stress, hence building muscle.

Squats are a critical component of your muscle-building routine. Additionally, they work out the entire body.

Squats, deadlifts, barbell rows, bench presses, and dips should all be included in your fitness plan. This would provide an opportunity to work out the entire body.

A newbie requires additional time to recover from fitness routines. Appropriate sleep, rest, nutrition, and water to drink are necessary.

Your diet should include a suitable amount of protein, carbohydrates, vegetables, fat, and fruit. They contain vitamins and minerals that will assist you in recovering much more quickly.

Consume more food to gain weight. Additionally, meals should be spread evenly throughout the day. Protein should also be a part of your diet. They are critical in assisting you in maintaining and building muscle mass.

However, the most critical aspect to consider is perseverance. Do not surrender.

www.ingramcontent.com/pod-product-compliance
Lightning Source LLC
LaVergne TN
LVHW050601160826
845677LV00011B/2401

9798809924436